TUBERCULOSIS

AND ITS

PREVENTION

TUBERCULOSIS

AND ITS

PREVENTION

STEFAN GRZYBOWSKI, M.D., F.R.C.P.

Professor of Medicine
University of British Columbia, Canada

WARREN H. GREEN, INC.

St. Louis, Missouri, U.S.A.

Published by

WARREN H. GREEN, INC.
8356 Olive Blvd.
Saint Louis, Missouri, 63132 U.S.A.

ISBN No. 87527-198-7

Printed in the United States of America

TO MY

WIFE AND CHILDREN

PREFACE

"If preventable — why not prevented?" These words were uttered by King Edward VII about tuberculosis at the beginning of this century, yet some sixty or seventy years later there is still a need for a book updating our knowledge about this disease.

Tuberculosis is still a tremendous problem in the world today with an estimated ten million positive sputum cases of the disease arising in the world population every year. Tuberculosis has always been associated with poverty and it is not surprising therefore that this disease is much more prevalent in the poorer developing areas of the world than in the richer western countries. Yet, even in these countries, there are groups of population with high rates, such as American and Canadian Indians or inhabitants of our city ghettos.

This book is directed towards the medical readers both in the developed and developing countries. In order to truly prevent disease one has to understand not only the practical clinical aspects of diagnosis and treatment but must also have some insight into the more fundamental knowledge of the disease. The chapters on natural history review our current understanding of these areas. They deal with risk of infection and both the quantitative and temporal aspects of the relationship of infection to disease; the risk of developing the disease once infected, varies in different populations and the "timetable of tuberculosis" shows that different forms of disease occur at different intervals after infection. Explanation is suggested why in many instances tuberculosis, which not so many years ago was a disease of young women, now has become a disease predominantly of older men.

Various diagnostic tools at our disposal are discussed next. The value as well as the limitation of tuberculin test are discussed, as well as the influence of atypical mycobacterial infection on tuberculin sensitivity. Of other diagnostic tools the place of chest x-ray is considered as well as that of bacteriology. The importance of bacteriological investigation is emphasized; here like in so many other aspects of tuberculosis the western world owes a debt to developing countries and particularly to India where many excellent studies on tuberculosis have been done in the recent past.

The most important single preventive measure in this disease is early diagnosis and thorough treatment of the infectious cases; this results in the diminution of the risk of infection in the community. Case finding programs are important. In the developed countries with low rates of tuberculosis such programs should be mainly directed to special "high risk" groups and can utilize chest x-ray and tuberculin test. In some of the developing countries the most effective case finding program is by microscopic sputum examination of patients with productive cough.

Effective treatment of tuberculosis is possible under all economic circumstances. The secret is to prescribe adequate regimens and to secure compliance of patients.

The two specific preventive programs — BCG vaccination and chemoprophylaxis are considered in detail. In spite of the fact that in most countries, only one of these measures is widely used with almost complete exclusion of the other, these two measures are quite compatible.

Tuberculosis is declining steadily but slowly in most countries. This decline can be greatly accelerated by awareness and understanding of this disease among health professionals. It is hoped that this book will in a small measure contribute towards achieving the goal of a more rapid decline and eventual eradication of tuberculosis.

ACKNOWLEDGMENT

The author is deeply grateful to Dr. E.A. Allen, his life-long friend and colleague in tuberculosis research, for his helpful and stimulating criticism of this book and to Miss Elaine Dorken, P.H.N., for her assistance.

CONTENTS

TUBERCULOSIS

AND ITS

PREVENTION

CHAPTER I

NATURAL HISTORY OF TUBERCULOSIS IN AN INDIVIDUAL

PRIMARY TUBERCULOUS INFECTION

The first encounter of an individual with tubercle bacilli is the most important event in the natural history of tuberculosis. It is this event that sets the stage for possible future development of tuberculous disease. Fortunately, infection with tubercle bacilli does not usually lead to disease. At the turn of the century, for instance, practically all, if not all children living in large cities of Europe were infected with tubercle bacilli. This infection caused disease in many; however, the majority remained free of tuberculous disease throughout their life span; were it not so, mankind would have been wiped out by tubercle bacilli a long time ago.

Tubercle bacillus can therefore be considered as a somewhat reluctant pathogen, causing disease only in a minority of those infected. This risk of disease varies among different people of the world according to how recently in history people or a race become exposed. It has been estimated that in Caucasians infected with tubercle bacilli, some five to ten percent develop disease sometime in their lifetime. In races which have met the tubercle bacillus relatively recently, morbidity is much greater; for instance in Eskimos this risk of disease is appreciably higher around 40 percent. Yet, the tubercle bacillus is obviously much more pathogenic than its cousins — "atypical" mycobacteria — which cause disease only in a fraction of one percent of those infected.

What are the factors which determine why one infected individual develops disease and may indeed die of tuberculosis, while in another tuberculous infection is an insignificant event causing him no trouble whatsoever? Not all these factors are known and the significance of some is controversial. They can conveniently be considered under three headings: Seed, Host and Accident.

A. The Seed

1. Virulence — Tubercle bacilli vary in virulence; there is good evidence for instance, that tubercle bacilli predominant in India are less virulent than those encountered in Europe. We also know that some tubercle bacilli rendered highly resistant to Isoniazid become less virulent. Beyond these two well established facts little is known about the differences, and possible changes in virulence of tubercle bacilli. Most authorities discount virulence as an important factor in epidemiology of tuberculosis; yet we should perhaps keep an open mind and explore the possibility that virulence may be changing in time and that this could explain occasional unexpected epidemiological findings, such as very low morbidity among recently infected unvaccinated individuals in the recent BCG trial in India.

Certainly in the laboratory we can affect the virulence of tubercle bacilli; the best example is the development of BCG vaccine, from virulent bovine tubercle bacilli, to an attenuated state. The loss of virulence associated with the development of high degrees of Isoniazid resistance is particularly interesting when one considers that most atypical mycobacteria show very low virulence and are usually resistant to antimicrobial agents.

2. Dose — The number of bacilli received at primary infection is important; this is shown for instance by studies on contacts of active cases of tuberculosis. These studies show that contacts of potent sources of infection — those with positive sputum smears, are not only more frequently infected, but are also more "dangerously" infected, than is the case in contacts of patients whose sputum is positive on culture only(1). In other words, the rate of disease among infected contacts of smear positive cases is greater than among infected contacts of culture positive cases.

Some authorities believe that only one or at the most a few bacilli are always responsible for infection; this belief was strengthened by the work of Riley(2) who has shown that tiny respirable droplets can contain only a very small number of bacilli. Yet, both epidemiological and experimental evidence clearly reveals the importance of the dose of bacilli received at primary infection.

B. The Host

1. Natural Resistance — It has already been pointed out that infected Eskimos develop disease more frequently than infected Caucasians. This is, in part, because the Eskimos as a race encountered the tubercle bacillus within the past 100 years(68), whereas Caucasians have been exposed for many centuries. This resulted in the augmentation of natural (native) immunity (herd resistance) in Caucasians; the more susceptible individuals died of their disease in the past, while the more resistant survived and multiplied. Tuberculosis in races with low natural resistance is often thought to be associated with certain peculiar clinical features such as pronounced lymph node enlargement and frequency of pericarditis. Curiously, these clinical features were not observed in Eskimos, in whom the clinical picture seemed identical to that seen in the Caucasian patients. The fact that Eskimos and North American Indians show a greater risk of reactivations (relapses) than similarly treated white patients, is possibly another manifestation of the same factor — lower natural resistance(3,4).

2. Age and Sex — The age at which individuals become infected with tubercle bacilli is of great importance. Infants and very young children are prone to develop disseminated hematogenous forms of tuberculosis, particularly dreaded meningitis. On the other hand, the frequency of post-primary pulmonary tuberculosis is lower in children infected in the first few years of life, even when followed up into adult life, than that seen in infected adolescents and adults(5). Primary tuberculous infection acquired in adolescence, if it progresses to disease, most commonly leads to post-primary pulmonary tuberculosis within months; although of course this form of the disease may occur many years, even many decades after primary infection but the risk diminishes with the passage of time. Sex is also of importance as shown by the fact that when tuberculous infection was almost universal, it was the young women who most frequently suffered and died of this disease; this pattern is also clearly apparent at present when morbidity rate is calculated among infected segment of population(6,7).

C. The Accident

"Pathological accident" plays a part in determining the fate of an infected individual. In a child with primary tuberculosis, an affected gland may perforate into a blood vessel, causing overwhelming hematogenous spread of disease, while in another child, a similar gland may perforate into a bronchus, giving rise to the rather benign complication of "epituberculosis." Primary foci which happen to be situated in upper and posterior areas of the lungs are more likely to give rise to post-primary tuberculosis than similar foci situated elsewhere in the lungs(8).

EFFECTS OF PRIMARY INFECTION

Primary tuberculous infection has two effects:
(1) Detrimental to the host by planting the seed of future disease in the lungs and other organs;
(2) Beneficial to the host by providing him with strong immunity against further infection from outside (acquired resistance).

1. Hematogenous Dissemination — is the most important way of seeding tubercle bacilli to various organs of the body; these foci take different durations of time in different organs to mature into overt disease. There is some evidence that hematogenous dissemination may occur in the course of almost every primary infection; however, clinically significant dissemination is less frequent. Hematogenous dissemination usually occurs within a few months of primary infection, and this is when the most obvious acute form of disease due to dissemination — miliary tuberculosis is usually seen. However, hematogenous spread may occur much later from previously established pulmonary or extra-pulmonary foci; this may, for instance, happen as a result of treatment with corticosteroids.

2. Acquired Resistance — Primary infection results in strong acquired resistance against any further infection. Many observations attesting to this will be mentioned in various places of this book. They will include such varied observations as the fact that heavy exposure to tuberculous infections takes much less of a toll of those who were initially tuberculin positive than of those who were tuberculin negative. It is also now proven conclusively that primary infection with bovine tubercle bacilli exerts a potent protective influence insofar as the development of pulmonary tuberculosis is concerned. Furthermore, previously infected nurses who develop pulmonary tuberculosis when looking after patients with drug resistant tubercle bacilli, usually have sensitive organisms arising from their original infection.

Resistance acquired from infections with virulent bacilli, be it human or bovine, is much stronger than that acquired as a result of infection with atypical mycobacteria or artificial infection with attenuated strain of bovine bacilli (BCG vaccination).

TIME TABLE OF TUBERCULOSIS

As has already been emphasized, the single most important event in the natural history of tuberculosis, is primary infection. Various forms of tuberculous disease tend to arise at certain times following primary infection. The credit for this observation goes to Wallgren who, in 1948, described it under the heading of "Time Table of Tuberculosis"(9). Table 1 represents a modified outline of this Time Table.

TABLE I

TIME TABLE OF TUBERCULOSIS

Incubation Period—6 weeks (3–8 weeks)	Tuberculin conversion	100%
	Primary illness	30%
	Erythema nodosum	5%

Complications and Sequelae	Usual Time After Conversion	Frequency in Caucasians
1. Epituberculosis	0–6 months	5–10% of younger children
2. Pleural effusion	2–9 months	5–10% adults, adolescents and older children
3. Miliary and meningitis	2–9 months	5–10% of children under two; later dropping to 1%
4. Extrapulmonary tuberculosis		
(a) cervical lymphadenitis	Few months–many years later	
(b) skeletal tuberculosis	First few years	
(c) genito-urinary tuberculosis	Many years later	
5. Post-primary pulmonary tuberculosis	At and after puberty	10% in recently infected adolescents 4% in those infected in earlier childhood

It will be seen that most of the complications and sequelae tend to occur at well defined times following primary infection. Most of the cases of epituberculosis occur within the first six months following tuberculin conversion; tuberculous pleural effusion (''primary effusion'') also occurs quite early. On the other hand, genito-urinary tuberculosis is usually a very late sequel; some Scandinavian studies suggest that the average period from infection is somewhere between 20 to 30 years. Post-primary pulmonary tuberculosis (''chronic pulmonary tuberculosis'' — ''phthisis'') does not have a constant time relationship to infection, but when the latter takes place in childhood then this form of disease tends to occur at and after puberty(5). The frequency of occurrence of each of the sequelae is shown in Table I. These figures are based on studies of white children hospitalized for primary tuberculosis(8,9), and there is good evidence that these percentages are much higher among children of other races. For instance a study of North American Indian children the frequency of ''sequelae'' was five times higher and mortality nine times higher

TABLE 2

COMPARISON OF COMPLICATIONS OF PRIMARY TUBERCULOSIS IN INDIAN AND WHITE CHILDREN—SEVEN YEAR FOLLOW-UP PERIOD

	Did well	Subsequent TB Morbidity	Mortality
White Children (High Wood—486)	437 (90%)	49 (10%)	6 (1%)
Indian Children (B.C.—165)	84 (51%)	81 (49%)	18 (11%)

than among similarly studied white children(10). There are some suggestions that the risks of various sequelae following primary infection may be lower now in the white children than indicated in Table I; this would appear reasonable if the dose of bacilli received at primary infection matters. With the declining risk of tuberculous infection in the community seen in most countries of the world, one would expect that those infected receive, on the average, a smaller number of bacilli, and subsequently show lower morbidity. Such an hypothesis is in keeping with the findings of studies of contacts of active cases of tuberculosis which show that infected contacts of smear positive cases ("large dose of bacilli") show higher morbidity than the contacts infected by smear negative cases ("smaller dose of bacilli")(1).

Table I makes it clear that the type of complication or sequelae is very much dependent on the age of the infected child, thus, infants and very young children show a high rate of developing epituberculosis; and infants have a high risk of developing serious hematogenous forms of disease — miliary spread, and tuberculous meningitis. When infection occurs later in adolescence or young adult life, tuberculous pleural effusion becomes the most common complication. The risk of developing post-primary pulmonary tuberculosis is greatest if the infection is acquired at or after puberty; this risk is smaller in those who are infected in early childhood(5). It may be said that in old days when getting infected with tubercle bacilli during childhood was unavoidable, the "optimum" time to be infected was somewhere between five and ten years of age. At this age, the danger of miliary disease and meningitis has already appreciably receded; while at the same time, the risk of post-primary pulmonary tuberculosis was still significantly lower than that seen in those infected in adolescence.

This discussion is based primarily on the studies conducted on children and adolescents. Investigations conducted on young adults, particularly nurses(11), exposed to tuberculous infection, indicate that the risks of various forms of disease are generally similar to those seen in adolescence. There is, however, very little information on the risks of primary tuberculous infection when it is acquired after the age of thirty.

CHAPTER II

PRIMARY PULMONARY TUBERCULOSIS

For some six weeks (4 to 8) following primary infection with tubercle bacilli, the individual is clinically quite well, and if tuberculin tested during this period, the test is negative. At the end of this period, there is invariably tuberculin conversion — the test becomes positive and the degree of sensitivity is usually very high. The majority of the newly infected individuals are symptom-free at the time of conversion; some develop what Wallgren called "primary illness"(9). This is a flu-like condition; the main features are fever and unproductive cough. A much smaller proportion of infected individuals develop erythema nodosum(12); this, when tuberculous in origin, almost inevitably occurs at the time of tuberculin conversion. Scandinavians and northern Europeans are more prone to erythema nodosum than other races, whether caused by sarcoidosis, tuberculosis, or any other condition or drug.

Primary tuberculous infection results in the establishment of primary complex (Figure 1). This consists of a parenchymal lesion — "primary focus" — and of enlargement of the lymph nodes draining the affected area of the lung. While every pulmonary primary infection results in establishment of the primary complex, this is clearly visible in the chest radiographs only in a minority of infected individuals. This may be because the lesions are very small or because an appreciable part of the lung parenchyma and mediastinal lymph nodes is not visible in an ordinary radiological examination. Enlargement of hilar lymph nodes alone, without a visible primary focus is seen more frequently than both components of primary complex.

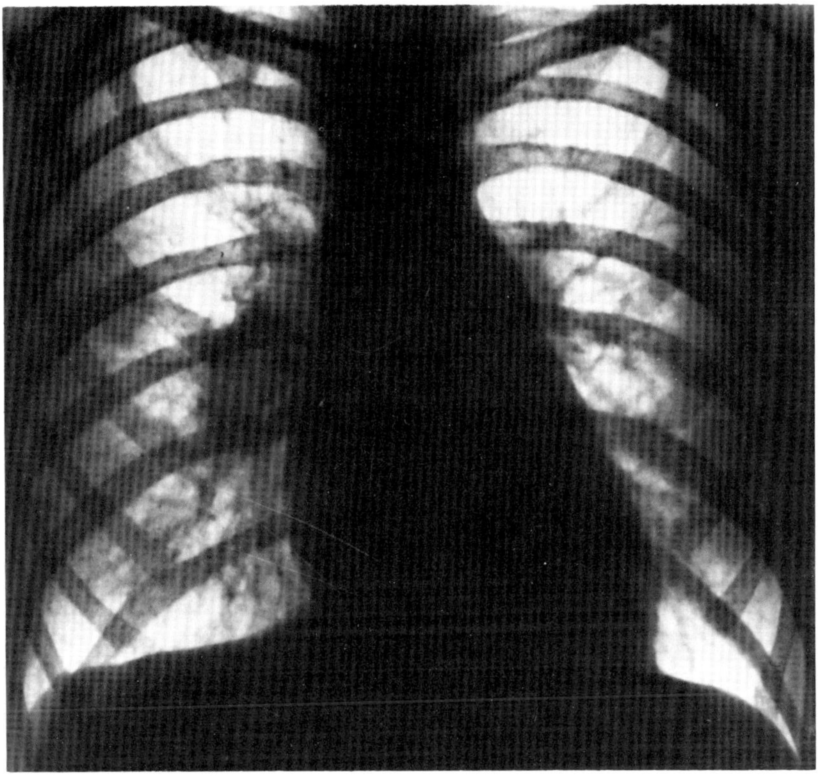

Figure 1. Primary complex—right lung in a 10-year-old girl.

Such enlargement is often somewhat uncertain as the lymph nodes in primary tuberculosis are seldom grossly enlarged, and the size of normal hilar shadows vary from individual to individual. Occasionally, right paratracheal nodes are enlarged as well as hilar nodes; enlargement of these nodes is of clinical significance as hematogenous forms of tuberculosis are most common in children with this finding(8).

It is customary to use the term primary pulmonary tuberculosis when there is a definite radiological abnormality consisting of a primary complex or enlargement of hilar glands alone; if no radiological abnormality is discernable in a recently infected individual, the term "recent convertor" is often used. While all recently infected individuals convert their tuberculin reaction from negative to positive, it should not be forgotten that primary tuberculous infection is only one of the causes of tuberculin conversion; this will be discussed fully later.

Uncomplicated primary pulmonary tuberculosis usually runs a very benign course. The primary lung focus which usually consists of a single density of less than 1 cm in diameter, diminishes in size over a period of months and often shows first signs of calcification during the second year following primary infection. Similarly, hilar nodes remain enlarged for a period of months and then gradually diminish in size; if calcification appears, it also begins to be radiologically discernable during the second year after primary infection; it becomes denser and better defined during the ensuing few years. It is of interest that calcification is more frequently seen in children infected by other household members (contacts) than in those infected elsewhere where the source of infection remains undiscovered(8). This is probably because household contacts are infected with a larger dose of tubercle bacilli causing more extensive caseation with subsequent calcification.

CHAPTER III

EPITUBERCULOSIS (SEGMENTAL LESIONS)

This is a common complication of primary tuberculosis, particularly in the first few years of childhood. The term, "lobar or segmental lesions" suggested at one time by the author and his colleagues did not achieve recognition, neither did such terms as "collapse consolidation" or "tuberculous perifocal pneumonia." Because of this, the time honored, though admittedly meaningless term of "epituberculosis"(13) is resurrected here. Very recently DeKock suggested the term lympho-bronchial tuberculosis. In this form of disease whole anatomical units of the lungs (lobes or bronchopulmonary segments) are involved and cast characteristic shadows on the chest x-ray. (Figures 2A, B, C) This condition is rather benign. Insofar as future tuberculous disease is concerned, the outlook for children with epituberculosis does not appear to be worse than for those with simple primary tuberculosis. In olden days when this was not realized, children with epituberculosis were frequently hospitalized for very prolonged periods, as the physicians erroneously applied to those young patients, the lesson they learned from looking after post-primary tuberculosis — the more extensive shadows, the worse the outlook. Later, surgical resection of these lesions became fashionable in some centres. With the introduction of antimicrobial therapy, the outlook for these young patients became excellent, although the evolution of the shadows has not been significantly affected.

There were numerous hypotheses relating to the pathogenesis of epituberculosis which are of historical interest; we now know that we are dealing here with bronchial obstruction with collapse or consolidation behind such obstruction. Bronchoscopic findings show mark-

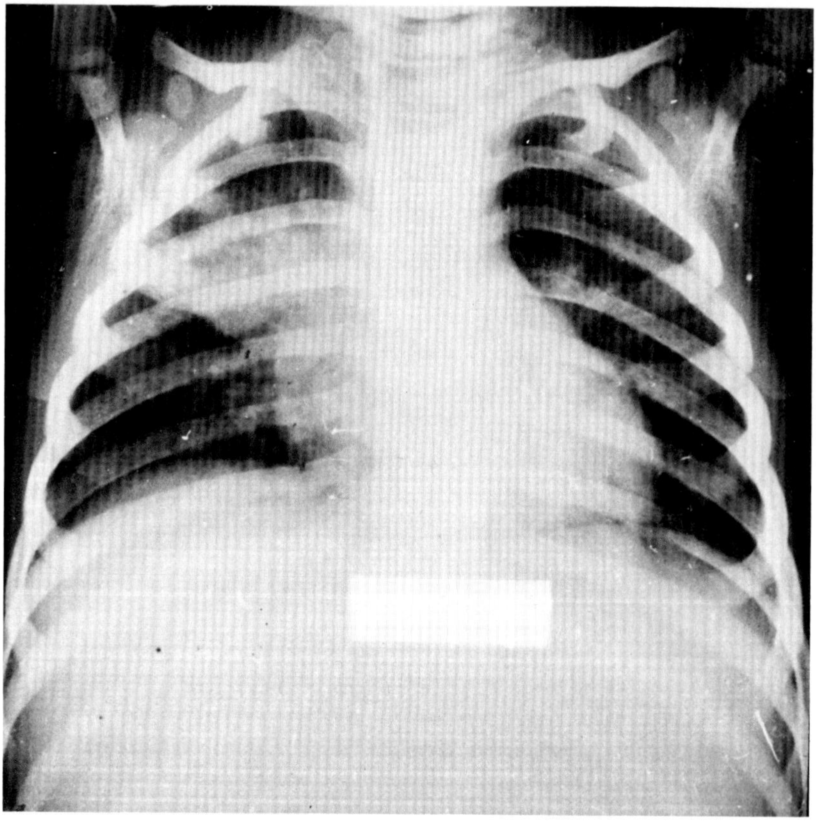

Figures 2A & B. Epituberculosis involving the anterior segment of the right upper lobe in a child age 5.

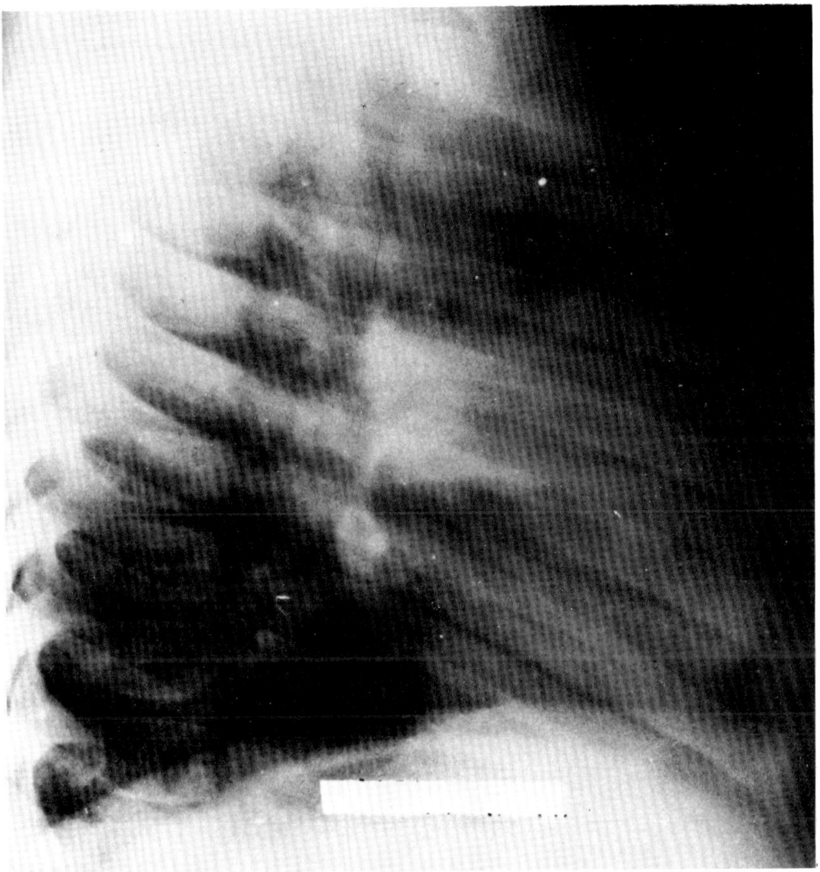

Figure 2B.

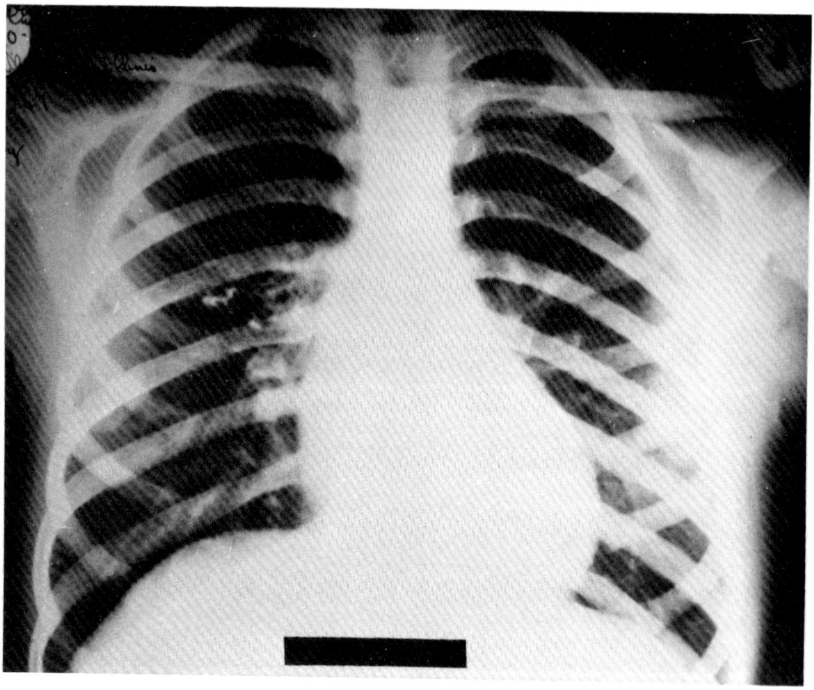

Figure 2C. Seven years later—typical end result with collapsed segment and calcification.

ed occlusion of the bronchi by the enlarged lymph nodes with frequent fistula formation and granulation tissue arising from the bronchial wall. The fact that bronchi of younger children are smaller and more pliable accounts for a higher frequency of these lesions in early childhood.

The pathological picture varies and may consist of: atelectasis, non specific pneumonia, multiple granulomas and caseation. This is understandable, as we are dealing here with bronchial stenosis or occlusion; and such factors as secondary infection, aspiration of the caseating material from a discharging lymph node as well as the possible presence of the primary focus in the affected segment all contribute.

Segmental lesions develop within the first few months after primary infection, occasionally they are seen as early as the time of tuberculin conversion. Very few of these lesions appear after six months has elapsed since infection; although, as will be discussed later, the resulting permanent bronchostenosis occasionally leads to reappearance of the shadow, sometimes years later — this is almost invariably precipitated by intercurrent respiratory infection.

There are often no symptoms whatsoever when these lesions first appear, although in the minority, the onset is heralded by high fever and cough.

Epituberculosis may affect any lobe or segment of the lung; however, the lesions involving the right middle lobe, anterior segment of the right upper lobe and of the left upper lobe or one of their sub-segments, are most common. Radiologically, the shadows of segmental lesions persist and tend to contract slowly over a period of many months. The usual end-result is a linear scar representing a collapsed scarred segment. (Figure 2C) Such a narrow linear scar is difficult to discern in the case of many segments, but is obvious when anterior segments of the right or left upper lobe are affected.

"NON-TUBERCULOUS" SEQUELAE OF EPITUBERCULOSIS

When bronchograms are done in children who have recovered from epituberculosis, bronchiectasis and bronchostenosis are very commonly seen; however, in most instances, the individual does not suffer from any symptoms. Symptomatic bronchiectasis may occur occasionally, particularly in a patient with lobar rather than segmental lesions, when either one of the lower lobes, or the right middle lobe are involved. Bronchostenosis, which is frequently seen in these cases, leads, at times to recurrent pneumonitis of the affected segment. This usually occurs in the course of respiratory infections, sometimes many years after recovery from tuberculosis. Such pneumonitis is often confused with a relapse of tuberculosis or if it occurs later in life, with carcinoma of the lung. At times, more severe pneumonia or even suppurative pneumonias may appear. This has been well described by Brock(14) as "post-tuberculous bronchostenosis of the right middle lobe" and has been known as Brock's syndrome or Right Middle Lobe Syndrome. Similar "syndromes" may occur in other segments which were initially affected by primary tuberculosis. Very occasionally, the calcification present in the lymph nodes or in the lung parenchyma ulcerates into the bronchus and may present as broncholiths.

The mainstay of treatment of epituberculosis are antimicrobials; this will be discussed later. No special treatment is necessary for most of these children and surgical interference is unwarranted unless there are severe symptoms resulting from bronchiectasis or bronchostenosis, such as repeated pneumonias, hemoptysis etc. "Prophylactic" surgery — resection of affected segments because the shadow does not resolve quickly enough or because bronchiectasis is present, in the absence of symptoms is unjustified. Children with epituberculosis, like those with simple primary tuberculosis, are not infectious and isolating them or barring them from attendance at school is not necessary.

CHAPTER IV

TUBERCULOUS PLEURAL EFFUSION

Tuberculous pleural effusion (primary pleural effusion) is the most common complication of primary tuberculous infection in older children, adolescents, and young adults. Studies indicate that this form of disease may occur in up to 10 percent of recently infected males and in a slightly lower proportion of recently infected females. The majority of cases occur within six months after primary infection. Occasionally, pleural effusion appears many years after primary infection; it then often complicates post-primary pulmonary tuberculosis, but may be the only manifestation of tuberculosis.

Pathogenesis of tuberculous pleural effusion is not completely understood, and probably more than one mechanism is involved. The fact that effusions usually occur on the same side as primary complex suggests that they are due to the direct extension of the tuberculous process to the pleura either from the primary focus or from the lymph node. However, pleural effusion may be a manifestation of miliary tuberculosis; this should be suspected when effusion is bilateral, or heterolateral to the primary complex.

Prognosis of patients with pleural effusion appears to be slightly worse than that of patients with simple primary tuberculosis. If untreated with antimicrobials, some 10 to 15 percent of these individuals develop post-primary pulmonary tuberculosis within the next 5 to 10 years and another 5 percent or so develop extra-pulmonary forms of the disease(15). Adequate antimicrobial therapy given at the time of pleural effusion substantially diminishes subsequent morbidity.

The presenting symptoms in most cases are fever and a typical pleural pain; there is also usually some unproductive cough. Depending on the amount of fluid, there are varying degrees of dyspnea. An uncommon presentation is a small hemoptysis.

Physical examination reveals the well-known signs of diminished movement, "stony" dullness, diminished breath sounds and occasionally aegophony. In early cases, pleural rub is heard.

Diagnosis is usually not difficult in the young subjects, as "idiopathic" pleural effusion associated with a positive tuberculin reaction should be considered tuberculous until proven otherwise. A thoracocentesis should always be done, for diagnosis and often for relief of dyspnea. The fluid is usually clear, but may be bloody. It has typical characteristics of an exudate with specific gravity over 1.016 and protein contents of over 3.5 grams. The fluid contains predominantly lymphocytes, but a few neutrophils and mesothelial cells are also seen; it should be remembered that the latter often look quite bizarre and this may occasionally lead to a false diagnosis of malignancy. With thorough bacteriological methods tubercle bacilli can be grown from the fluid quite frequently (up to 80% of cases); they are, however, infrequently seen on microscopy.

Needle biopsy of the pleura often shows caseating granulomata: a part of the biopsy material should always be sent for bacteriology. Glucose level in the effusion is almost invariably diminished.

Radiologically the picture of pleural effusion is quite characteristic when costal pleura is involved. Sub-pneumonic or other localized effusions are uncommon as a presenting feature when tuberculosis is the cause. Fluid absorbs slowly over a period of several weeks or a few months and commonly leaves permanent radiological obliteration of the costophrenic angle as evidence of previous effusion. Occasionally during resorption, absorption of fluid occurs unevenly in various parts of the pleural cavity and this sometimes results in localized pleural shadows which may simulate closely parenchymal lesions and become a source of worry to the medical attendant. This worry disappears with the disappearance of the abnormal shadow usually within a few weeks. Occasionally, the primary complex or one of its components are seen, particularly when fluid clears up.

CHAPTER V

MILIARY TUBERCULOSIS

Miliary tuberculosis is a manifestation of hematogenous dissemination which tends to occur early after the primary infection especially in infants. It may, however, occur much later as a result of dissemination from any of the previously established foci of the disease; such late dissemination may be the result of severe debilitating illness often in the presence of old age, alcoholism, malnutrition or corticosteroid treatment. In countries where tuberculous infection is still common and some 30 to 40 years ago in North America and Western Europe, the first of these mechanisms — dissemination following closely primary infection is frequent and the majority of cases of miliary tuberculosis occur in early childhood. Nowadays, in North America with the decline in the risk of tuberculous infection, late dissemination from secondary foci is seen more frequently and the majority of cases of miliary tuberculosis are seen in adults, often in the older age groups. In the latter setting the diagnosis is frequently missed.

In children dissemination probably occurs from either components of the primary complex — from primary focus or from the affected lymph node; likely the tuberculous lesion erodes the blood vessel wall and empties into its lumen. Children with miliary tuberculosis often show enlargement of the right paratracheal glands and children with primary tuberculosis who show paratracheal enlargement develop hematogenous forms of tuberculosis more often than those without such a finding. This suggests that blood dissemination may also occur through the lymphatic duct. In cases occurring late in the disease, a pulmonary or perhaps more often an extra-pulmonary focus erodes into a vessel. Miliary foci are scattered throughout the body, affecting lungs, liver, kidney, spleen, bone marrow, meninges and many other organs.

The clinical picture of miliary tuberculosis varies. Most cases present as "pyrexia of unknown origin". Cough, usually unproductive, may be present and there may also be a varying degree of dyspnea. Occasionally symptoms are mild.

Physical signs are often absent. However careful examination of the fundi may reveal miliary tubercles in a minority of patients. There may also be some generalized lymph node enlargement. Examination of the chest usually reveals no abnormality. In a few cases, there is hepato- and splenomegaly. Tuberculin test is usually positive although a larger dose (250 TU) may occasionally be necessary to elicit the reaction, as the degree of tuberculin sensitivity is often somewhat depressed in miliary tuberculosis. Chest x-ray characteristically shows a typical "snow-storm" appearance with small miliary nodules scattered throughout both lung fields (Figure 3). There may also be evidence of primary complex, of enlargement of paratracheal glands or of segmental lesions. However, it should not be forgotten that the chest x-ray is not infrequently normal. In a study of 100 consecutive children dying from tuberculosis in London, England, the author and his colleagues found that some 40 percent of children whose autopsy revealed miliary tuberculosis in the lungs had a normal chest x-ray a few days before death(8). Sputum is often absent and when present it is usually negative on smear examination.

Diagnosis of miliary tuberculosis may be difficult; in order to establish it definitely, biopsy of the lung, liver or bone marrow is sometimes necessary.

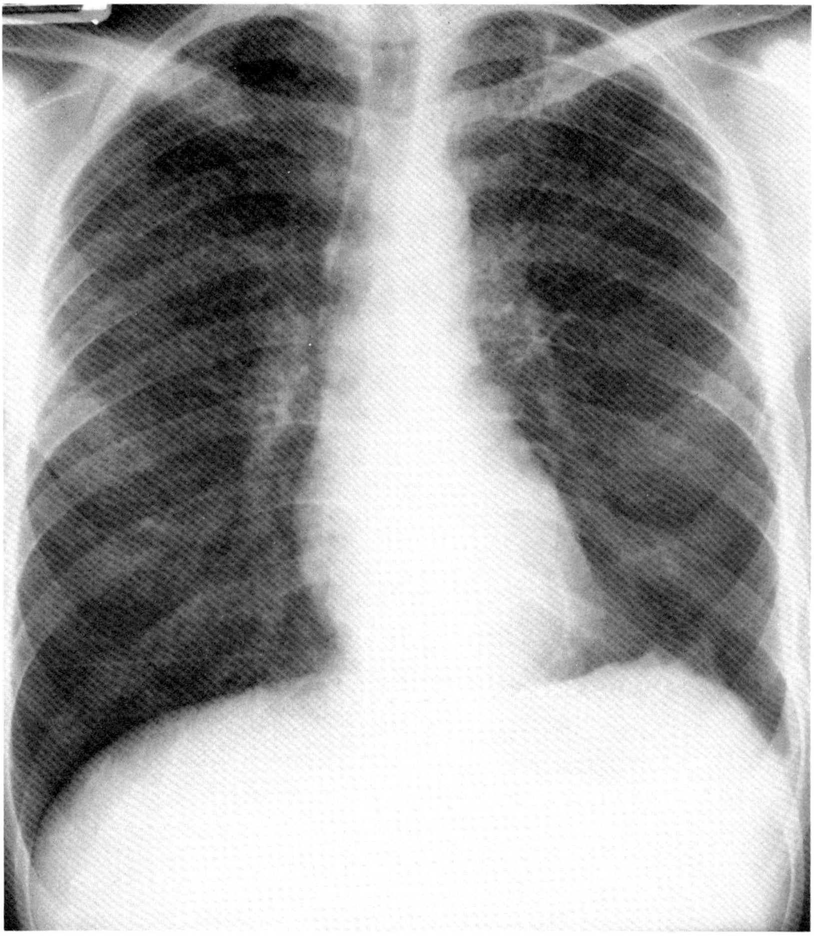

Figure 3. Miliary tuberculosis in a young man age 19.

CHAPTER VI

EXTRA THORACIC (EXTRA-PULMONARY) TUBERCULOSIS

Extra-thoracic tuberculosis still accounts for close to one-fifth of all cases of tuberculosis. In Canada, for instance, some 17 percent of total cases are accounted for by these forms of the disease. Only the most common or most serious forms will be discussed briefly here.

Study of the epidemiology of specific forms of extra-pulmonary tuberculosis is interesting. In a country such as Canada in which tuberculous infection has become uncommon, those forms of the disease which occur a long time after infection (e.g., genitourinary tuberculosis) are becoming relatively more frequent while those usually occurring early after infection (e.g., tuberculous meningitis) have become rather rare. There is racial predilection to certain forms of disease. People from Asia appear predisposed to tuberculous lympadenitis while those born in Southern Europe, particularly the Italians, are particularly prone to the development of genitourinary tuberculosis(16). Among black people of South Africa there is a striking incidence of tuberculous pericarditis often early after primary infection(17).

TUBERCULOUS MENINGITIS

Tuberculous meningitis is the most serious form of tuberculosis; it is the single most important form of tuberculous disease causing death in children. In a study of 100 consecutive deaths from tuberculosis in childhood occurring in London area (1948 to 1950) the author and his colleagues found that 86 of these 100 children under the age of 16 succumbed to meningitis(8). Today, deaths from tuberculosis among children are very uncommon but they are still almost invariably due to tuberculous meningitis.

In the pre-antimicrobial era, tuberculous meningitis was almost always fatal; now complete cure can be achieved if the diagnosis is made early; unfortunately many cases are diagnosed late and mental defect and other neurological deficits are common on "recovery." Tuberculous meningitis results from a blood dissemination of tubercle bacilli. About half of the cases have a clear-cut clinical and radiological picture of miliary tuberculosis often antedating the onset of meningitis by a period of a few weeks. It is possible that a small cortical tuberculoma arises as a result of blood dissemination (Rich's focus) and subsequently tubercle bacilli from this small lesion disseminate through the cerebro-spinal fluid.

In countries where tuberculous infection is still common, most cases of tuberculous meningitis arise in infants and young children occurring usually in the first six months following primary infection, although a number may occur during the second six month period. In countries where the risk of tuberculous infection has become very low, most of the relatively few cases of meningitis, like those of miliary tuberculosis arise through dissemination from a long established tuberculous focus, either pulmonary or extra-pulmonary, precipitated for instance by cortico-steroid therapy.

Tuberculous meningitis usually presents with classical symptoms of vomiting and headache. The mother may have noted a change in the child's disposition antedating these two symptoms by a few days, drowsiness and convulsions are common a little later. To these the presence of fever should be added particularly in cases starting as miliary tuberculosis. Occasionally there is a history of head injury preceeding immediately the onset of meningitis.

Classical signs of meningitis such as neck rigidity and Kernig's sign are often present but in earlier cases may be absent or only "slight" or "suggestive." Other signs include the presence of choroidal tubercles in a substantial minority of the cases particularly those associated with miliary tuberculosis. Enlargement of cervical glands and splenomegaly occur in a small number.

Because of the rather insidious onset and often indefinite physical signs early in the disease, there may be some delay in diagnosis; the majority of cases being diagnosed during second week of the illness.

Although tuberculin sensitivity is often depressed due to constitutional illness, most show a positive tuberculin reaction to the usual 5 TU dose and practically all of the remainder react to a large dose of tuberculin (250 TU). It is the author's practice when dealing with a patient suspected of having tuberculous meningitis to give 5 TU dose in one arm and 250 TU in another in order to save time.

Chest x-ray shows no obvious abnormality in about a quarter of the cases. When abnormality is present it most commonly consists of miliary mottling. There may however only be evidence of enlarged hilar nodes, of primary complex or of segmental lesions. Occasionally pleural effusion is present.

Examination of the cerebrospinal fluid is essential and should be done promptly on the first suspicion of meningitis. The fluid is usually under increased pressure; it is clear and shows slight elevation of protein, low glucose and an increased number of the cells consisting of both lymphocytes and polymorphs. It must be emphasized that absence of one of these findings does not negate the possibility of tuberculous meningitis; the author has seen the diagnosis missed because normal glucose level was erroneously thought to exclude the possibility of tuberculous etiology. Somewhat similar findings in the cerebrospinal fluid are seen in meningitis due to viruses, fungi and in meningitis carcinomatosa. Occasionally, a pellicle forms when the fluid has stood for a while and acid fast bacilli may be found in this pellicle. This is unfortunately uncommon, but tubercle bacilli are grown from the cerebrospinal fluid in the majority of cases. It is of course not justifiable to await the result of culture, as bacteriological confirmation would then arrive some weeks after the patient's demise. It is essential in the suspected case to commence antimicrobial treatment immediately while continuing the study of the patient.

TUBERCULOUS LYMPHADENITIS (TUBERCULOUS CERVICAL LYMPHADENITIS)

Tuberculous cervical lymphadenitis (scrofula) was at one time a very common form of extra-pulmonary tuberculosis as evidenced by the presence of characteristic scars in the necks of many older individuals.

Pathogenesis of this condition is most interesting. In the old days in many countries, most cases were due to infection with bovine tubercle bacilli acquired through drinking contaminated milk. In these cases, cervical adenitis represented a glandular component of the primary complex; the primary focus being situated usually in the tonsil. Although bovine infection caused a lot of suffering, it was preferable, in the old days, to be infected by bovine bacilli through the drinking of tuberculous milk than by human bacilli expectorated by a tuberculous patient. Bovine infection protected the individual from developing the most common and the most dreaded form of tuberculosis — pulmonary tuberculosis. This observation was originally made in 1886 and is known as Marfan's Law — "patients with scrofula do not develop phthisis"(18). Although this observation was not believed for many decades it was nevertheless correct as proven by studies in Scotland and Denmark. Infection with bovine tubercle bacilli is now very uncommon accounting for less than one percent of Canadian cases of lymphadenitis.

In most patients seen nowadays, tuberculous lymphadenitis is a complication of primary pulmonary infection with human tubercle bacilli. While there is a possibility that in some instances there is a direct lymphatic spread from mediastinal lymph nodes to the cervical nodes, in the great majority cervical adenitis is due to hematogenous dissemination from the primary complex in the lungs.

This form of disease, as has already been pointed out, is much more common in some races than in others. In the study of the author and his colleagues(10), cervical adenitis occurred in 2 percent of the white children with primary pulmonary tuberculosis while the corresponding figure for North American Indian children was 13 percent.

Recent studies in Canada on tuberculosis morbidity in various groups of immigrants have shown that tuberculous cervical adenitis is particularly common among immigrants from China, India and Philippines. This form of disease accounts for about 25 to 30 percent of total cases of tuberculosis in immigrants from these countries; the corresponding figure for the total Canadian cases of tuberculosis is 5 percent. Bovine infection is uncommon even in this group of persons from the Orient.

In Caucasian children under the age of 10 in British Columbia, Canada, cervical adenitis due to "atypical" mycobacteria is appreciably more common than that due to tubercle bacilli. Even so the total number of such cases is quite small. In individuals over the age of 10 and in young children of other racial backgrounds, "atypical" mycobacterial adenitis is practically unknown.

Clinical manifestation of tuberculous cervical adenitis is the development of a lump or lumps in the neck. This is usually not accompanied by any constitutional symptoms although occasionally fever may be present. In the minority of cases, active or inactive tuberculosis of other organs is present. Tuberculin test is invariably positive except in cases due to atypical mycobacteria. In those the usual test with 5 TU is usually negative although sometimes may be weakly positive. Simultaneous testing with antigens derived from atypical mycobacteria particularly with PPD-Gause and PPD-Battey is diagnostically helpful in such cases showing larger reactions to these antigens than those elicited by PPD-S (tuberculin). Diagnosis is frequently established by biopsy of the affected gland; when this is submitted for culture the result is usually positive. Unfortunately the entire excised specimen is often placed in preserving fluid and in these cases one has to be content with the histological findings of caseating granuloma.

Investigation of these cases with a chest radiograph is obviously mandatory; careful search for tuberculosis at other extra-pulmonary sites should also not be neglected.

Tuberculous cervical adenitis may occur within the first months after primary tuberculous infection; it may, however, occur later although most of the new cases are probably confined to the first few years. This form of disease appears to respond to antimicrobial therapy rather more slowly than many other forms, and relapses appear to occur more frequently even following "adequate" chemotherapy. Surgical drainage or resection is occasionally indicated particularly when caseating material in the glands liquifies and there is a threat of sinus formation. There is no longer any place for the radical block dissection of tuberculous glands.

TUBERCULOSIS OF BONES AND JOINTS

This is still a fairly common form of tuberculous disease; in Canada it constitutes at present 2.6 percent of all active tuberculosis(19). It is often diagnosed after very considerable delay resulting in unnecessarily prolonged suffering and often permanent disability. The late diagnosis of tuberculosis of bones and joints is surprising as the majority of these cases show other evidence of tuberculous disease such as history of previous tuberculosis, often at the same site, or of co-existing active or inactive tuberculosis of the lungs or of other extra-pulmonary sites. The vertebral column particularly the lumbar and more rarely cervical spine is frequently affected (tuberculous spondylitis; Pott's Disease). It is relatively easy to distinguish these cases radiologically from the more common neoplastic involvement of vertebrae as intervertebral disks tend to be destroyed by tuberculosis while neoplasms tend to be restricted to bodies of the vertebrae. It is however not possible to radiologically distinguish tuberculosis from osteomyelitis of another kind, e.g., that due to staphylococci, brucella, typhoid, etc. The most dreaded sequela, that of paraplegia and of permanent deformity, should not happen if the diagnosis is made relatively early and treatment prescribed. The treatment consists of antimicrobial therapy and appropriate immobilization. The role of surgery in this form of disease has been rendered uncertain by recent international studies(20).

Tuberculous arthritis is almost as common as tuberculosis spondylitis. One joint is invariably affected, usually hip or knee although any joint may become the site of disease. Diagnosis is established by synovial biopsy and bacteriological examination of the synovial fluid.

GENITOURINARY TUBERCULOSIS

Genitourinary tuberculosis occurs late in the course of the natural history of tuberculosis. Studies in Scandinavia have revealed that in most instances manifestations of this form of the disease occur many years after primary infection. It is, therefore, not surprising that it becomes relatively more prominent in populations where the risk of tuberculous infection has receded to low levels. In such countries, genitourinary tuberculosis is the most common form of extra-pulmonary disease seen; in Canada, for instance, it accounts for just over 7 percent of the total cases of tuberculosis (41 percent of nonrespiratory cases).

The common sites affected are kidneys, ureters and bladder, epididymis in males and fallopian tubes and endometrium in females.

Detailed discussion of the clinical manifestations of tuberculosis of these various organs is beyond the scope of this book. Suffice it to say that renal tuberculosis frequently presents as sterile pyuria or hematuria; epididymitis as local swelling, and tuberculous salpingitis as sterility. As in other forms of tuberculosis, the tuberculin test is of appreciable diagnostic value as it is usually positive; however, a negative reaction does not exclude tuberculosis but simply renders it less likely in the differential diagnosis. Thorough bacteriological examination of urine in renal tuberculosis and of biopsy material and curettings in genital tuberculosis is often rewarded by success. In 90 percent of the cases the result is positive. It should be remembered that findings of acid fast bacilli on microscopic examination of urine may be misleading as saprophytic mycobacteria are frequently found.

CHAPTER VII

POST-PRIMARY PULMONARY TUBERCULOSIS

This is by far the most important form of tuberculosis. It accounts for the majority of total active cases reported in any country; in Canada, for instance, this form accounts for 70 percent of all active tuberculosis. It is also the only form of the disease which is infectious, providing thereby the means by which tuberculosis can perpetuate itself in a community.

The importance of this form of the disease is illustrated by the fact that in common language the word "tuberculosis" means this form of disease. Synonyms of the preferred term "post-primary pulmonary tuberculosis" are phthisis, consumption, and adult-type of tuberculosis. Pulmonary tuberculosis is the most common cause of death from this disease in adults. This form of the disease is infrequently seen in children and in those infected in early childhood it tends to appear at the age of puberty, somewhat earlier in girls than in boys.

The pathogenesis of post-primary pulmonary tuberculosis has been for many decades a subject of considerable controversy which possibly will never be settled. There are those who, like the author, believe that "endogenous reinfection" is the common mechanism through which most cases of this disease develop. "Endogenous reinfection" is a rather clumsy term implying reactivation of dormant infection under certain circumstances. Such circumstances may be stress, puberty, corticosteroid therapy, undernutrition, etc. Post-primary disease is particularly liable to develop if the lesion containing living tubercle bacilli is situated in the upper and dorsal parts of the lung which are particularly vulnerable to this disease. Such a lesion may be a primary focus but more commonly are apical hematogenous foci — the so-called "Simon Foci," resulting from early hematogenous dissemination(21).

The proponents of "exogenous reinfection" believe that most cases of post-primary pulmonary tuberculosis arise from a second infection acquired from an outside source. They hold that bacilli from outside are implanted in allergic tissues and that this causes an acute reaction similar to Koch's phenomenon, leading to caseation and cavitation.

This dispute between "endogenists" and "exogenists" is obviously not without practical implications; if proponents of exogenous reinfection were to be right such preventive measures as chemoprophylaxis would be pointless and BCG vaccination should indeed be harmful.

Localization of the lesions is usually quite characteristic (Figure 4). Upper and posterior parts of the lungs tend to be affected, the most commonly affected site being posterior segment of the right upper lobe, followed by the posterior sub-segment of the apicoposterior segment of the left upper lobe. Apical segments of the lower lobes are also frequent sites of this disease. In advanced stages of the disease, both lungs may be extensively affected, but usually, though not invariably one of the bases is spared. Curiously, in diabetes and in immunosuppressed subjects this characteristic localization of pulmonary tuberculosis is not always seen, the lesions may occur anywhere in the lungs. Spread in post-primary pulmonary tuberculosis is almost invariably through the bronchi to other parts of the lungs: hematogenous spread is very uncommon.

The lesions tend to caseate and subsequently liquefy with the development of cavities. In contradistinction to most other forms of tuberculosis the bacterial population tends to be very large. It has been estimated for instance that a cavity of about four to six cm. in diameter contains about 10^8–10^9 bacilli.

Clinical Features

Symptoms of post-primary pulmonary tuberculosis can be considered under three headings: respiratory, constitutional and those due to complications.

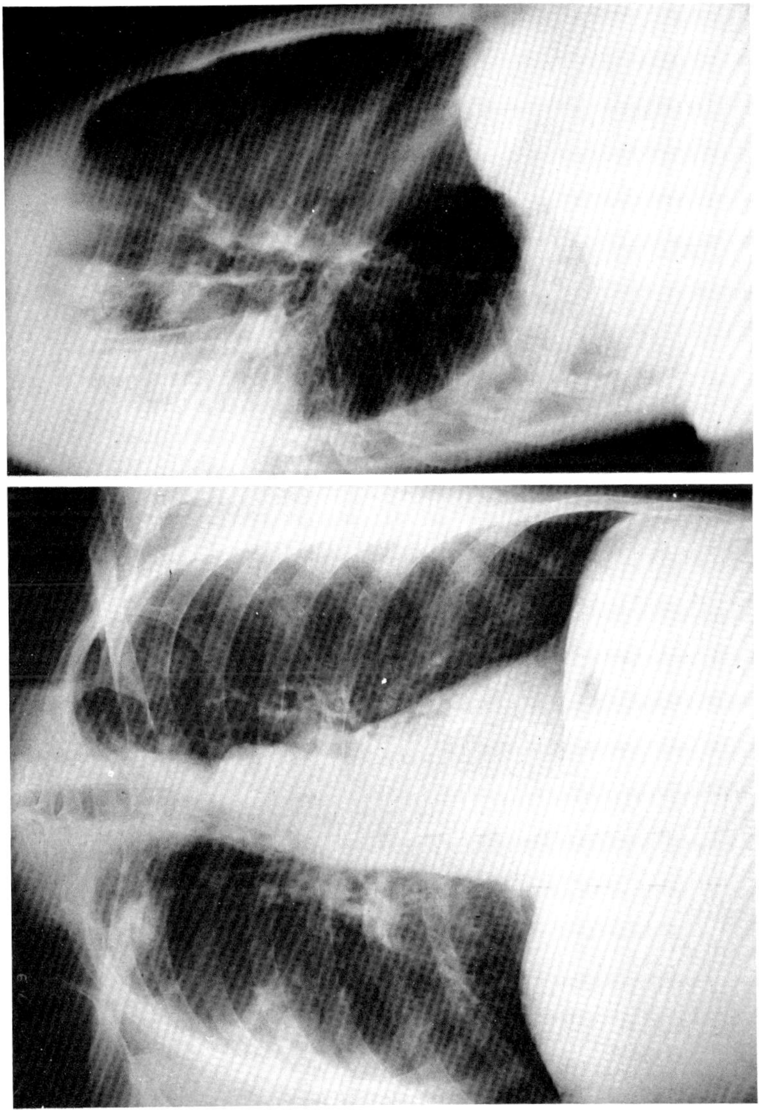

Figure 4. Post-primary tuberculosis; typical radiological appearance and localization.

Among respiratory symptoms cough predominates and is occasionally quite severe and irritating; it is usually productive of sputum which may be mucoid or mucopurulent. The most common cause of cough and sputum in the western world is of course chronic bronchitis due to cigarette smoking and to occupational and environmental pollution. However, in India with a much lower prevalence of bronchitis and much higher incidence of tuberculosis, 1 out of every 12 people with chronic productive cough has tubercle bacilli in his sputum. Hemoptysis is not very common in tuberculosis and usually consists of "staining of sputum." Very occasionally hemoptysis is quite severe and very infrequently it is fatal; in the latter cases hemoptysis is often due to the rupture of a small aneurysm in the cavity wall — the so-called Rasmussen aneurysm. Shortness of breath on exertion is usually not a noticeable symptom in the early stages. It may, however, be quite severe in extensive cases or those complicated by spontaneous pneumothorax. Chest pain of a pleuritic nature is relatively uncommon in this form of disease.

Constitutional symptoms consist of lassitude which is sometimes quite severe although in most cases the patient simply complains of feeling unwell. Loss of weight is frequent and there is sometimes spontaneous complaint of feeling hot and feverish. Night sweats, a time honoured symptom of tuberculosis, are actually relatively infrequent. Occasionally, particularly in young adults, the constitutional symptoms may simulate those of thyrotoxicosis.

Symptoms due to complications are relatively infrequent. In the past, when the diagnosis was often made very late in the course of the disease the patient may have presented with glossitis, laryngitis, enteritis or fistula-in-ano. Tuberculous glossitis is characterized by a painful ulcer on the edge of the tongue. Laryngitis often presents with hoarseness and pain, and enteritis with diarrhea. Fistula-in-ano is still a somewhat more common presentation of tuberculosis. These forms of disease are due to swallowing of sputum containing a very large number of tubercle bacilli.

History of contact with a case of tuberculosis, either recently or remotely, is common and should always be carefully enquired into.

Physical signs are often absent or are quite subtle, particularly when disease is not very extensive. In such cases, on inspection, one may observe a slight delay of movement in the upper portion of one side of the chest. Such "lagging" of movement is best observed with the physician standing behind the sitting patient with both hands overlying the patient's clavicles and observing the movement of the hands with respiration. Slight deviations of the trachea are also frequent. While Horner's syndrome is never caused by tuberculosis, there is occasionally dilatation of the pupil on the homolateral side probably due to irritation of the homolateral sympathetic fibers. Finger clubbing is not a sign of tuberculosis, it is, however, very occasionally seen in advanced cases. Fine crepitations heard over apices particularly after cough (post-tussive crepitations) are relatively common; listening for post-tussive crepitations was a routine way of screening recruits for tuberculosis in the First World War.

In advanced cases, almost any abnormal physical sign described in the examination of the chest may be elicited, although even here the radiological extent of the disease may be much greater than one would suspect from physical examination. Amphoric breath sounds are sometimes heard over cavities.

The unreliability of physical signs is well illustrated by the following story about the first chest x-ray taken in Edinburgh Royal Infirmary. A senior physician was doing rounds with the usual retinue of young doctors and students. He examined the chest of a new admission and said — "this man has a large cavity in the right apex." One of the registrars (residents) replied — "he just had an x-ray. Indeed he has a cavity but it is in the left apex." The undaunted chief responded — "I have always said that those new-fangled ideas are no good".

Laboratory investigations include three specific ones: tuberculin test, chest x-ray, and sputum bacteriology. These are considered in detail elsewhere in this book but certain practical aspects are discussed below:

1) ***Tuberculin Test:*** Usually Mantoux test with 5 TU of PPD-S or equivalent is used. Most patients with pulmonary tuberculosis show a clear cut positive reaction with a mean diameter of somewhere between 15 and 20 mm. However, about 20 percent show reactions below 10 mm. In one of our studies(22), reactions between 5 and 9 mm accounted for 7 percent; 4 percent had induration below 5 mm while 9 percent no measurable reaction whatsoever — 0 mm.

In some institutions it is customary to test with a smaller dose of tuberculin, e.g., 1 TU. This is done to avoid large reactions. This practice is unnecessary as even a very large reaction is seldom very painful, and inflammation usually settles within a day or two. The disadvantage of this practice is that occasionally the second test gets forgotten and a negative reactor to 1 TU is considered to be a non-reactor. Actually, for diagnosis of tuberculous disease it would be more rational to use a somewhat stronger dose than 5 TU in order to diminish the number of false negatives.

Early in this century tuberculin was used extensively, not only for the diagnosis, but for treatment. It is interesting to recall that at times a large dose of tuberculin or even an ordinary dose was purposely given subcutaneously; causing systemic reaction with fever as well as perifocal reaction(23). It has been apparently a practice in certain centres in the early 1900's to use tuberculin in such a way for diagnosis. It was felt for instance that eliciting perifocal reaction was a good test to use in tuberculosis of the joints. When following injection of tuberculin there was fever and the affected joint swelled up, the diagnosis was confirmed. To the author's knowledge nobody had used tuberculin perifocal reaction in investigation of solitary lung densities, and this may be worth trying.

2) ***Chest x-ray:*** is a time honoured tool in the diagnosis of pulmonary tuberculosis. The radiological appearances are often very highly suggestive though they are never absolutely pathognomonic. Lesions of post primary tuberculosis are often bilateral and have a strong tendency to specific localization in the upper and posterior portions of the lung (Figure 4). Not infrequently there are scattered calcifications in the neighbourhood of softer looking shadows. There is also a frequent cavity formation. It has been well documented that typical localization of tuberculous lesions is less commonly seen among diabetics. These patients' tuberculous lesions (and the juvenile diabetics are prone to this disease) may occur anywhere in the lungs and not infrequently the lower and more anterior parts of the lung are chiefly affected (e.g., right middle lobe or lingula). The reason for this peculiarity of localization of tuberculous lesions among diabetics is unknown (Figure 5).

3) ***Bacteriological examination of the sputum:*** This is the most important diagnostic tool in pulmonary tuberculosis. The vast majority

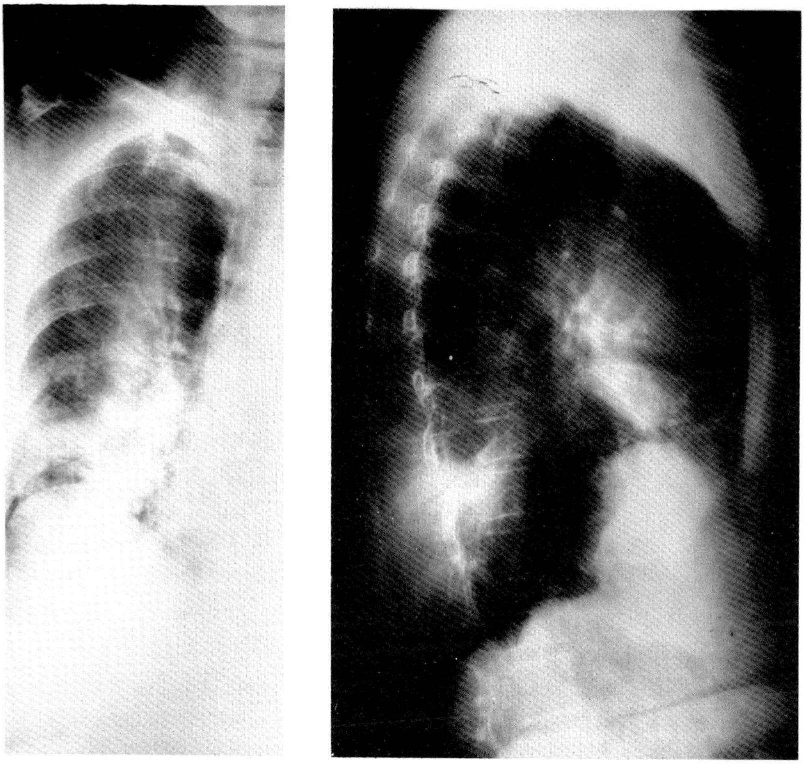

Figure 5. Post-primary tuberculosis in the right lung of a diabetic; unusual anterior localization of lesion.

of cases of active pulmonary tuberculosis are bacteriologically confirmed. In Canada, for instance, slightly more than 50 percent of patients diagnosed to have post primary pulmonary tuberculosis have positive sputum smear and another 30 percent while negative on smear have positive cultures. Only some 20 percent are bacteriologically unconfirmed. In some other countries the rate of bacteriological confirmation is much lower (well below 50 percent). While this may indicate inadequate bacteriological examination it usually reflects the fact that abnormal x-ray shadows in many patients are due either to inactive tuberculosis or to non-tuberculous conditions and are mistakenly treated as tuberculosis.

If no sputum is available there are four well recognized methods of obtaining secretion for bacteriological examination. Sputum induction with 10 percent propylen glycol in saline is effective in producing an adequate specimen in some 75 percent who do not have any spontaneous sputum. Gastric lavage is a time honoured method which is quite effective; it should be remembered however that positive smears obtained from gastric lavage should be interpreted with caution as they may not represent tubercle bacilli. Laryngeal swabs are done extensively in certain clinics and are quite effective. None of these methods is as good as sputum examination and they should not be resorted to in patients able to produce a specimen of sputum. Lastly bronchial washings obtained from fiberoptic bronchoscopy constitute excellent material for bacteriology although local anaesthetic may kill the organisms.

Differential diagnosis of pulmonary tuberculosis extends over most of the respiratory diseases with radiological abnormalities. In older men, tuberculosis has frequently to be differentiated from lung cancer which is now in North America some two to three times more common than tuberculosis in that group. Tuberculosis must be proved by isolation of the organism and lung cancer by positive sputum cytology or by biopsy. It is helpful to remember that lung cancer is almost invariably a unilateral disease while tuberculosis often affects both lungs. It should also be remembered that occasionally these two diseases coexist.

The Course of Pulmonary Tuberculosis: In the pre-antibiotic era we were able to observe the natural course of post-primary pulmonary tuberculosis. Usually a small apical or sub-apical lesion appeared first; it may have healed on its own or progressed; spread was almost invariably bronchogenic. In general, the course was characterized by rather rapid spread of disease followed by period of slow healing. Sudden exacerbations followed by slow prolonged remissions are similar to, what is for instance seen in multiple sclerosis. The whole story has often taken years to unfold, occasionally the progress was faster, the evolution with relapses and improvements taking months rather than years. In some cases, on the other hand, the evolution of the disease took almost a lifetime. It was presumed from this that if we diagnosed a case of far advanced pulmonary tuberculosis the disease in a less advanced stage was present for months or a few years. This view has been challenged recently by Styblo(24) and

Meijer(25) who believe that most far-advanced cases arise quite rapidly so that the diagnosis could not have been made much earlier. There is no doubt that such cases, in whom extensive tuberculosis developed in a matter of weeks, do exist, however, in author's experience they are a minority.

CHAPTER VIII

CONDITIONS PREDISPOSING TO TUBERCULOSIS

It is well known that a variety of conditions predispose to development of tuberculosis. The important ones, among them, are:

1) ***Silicosis or Silica Exposure:*** There is little doubt that exposure to silica makes one more susceptible to development of tuberculosis or to non-tuberculous (''atypical'') mycobacterioses. The exact mechanism is uncertain, but this predisposition is irrefutable. In a study conducted by the author and his colleague(26) in a mining town in northern Ontario, it was found that fully one-third of all those with silicosis had positive sputum for tubercle bacilli sometime during their life. Although it has been well documented that there are cases of tuberculosis in silicotics in whom tuberculosis runs a very rapid acute course, this is certainly not true for the vast majority of cases of silicotuberculosis. Indeed, some of these patients seem to live in a sort of symbiosis with tubercle bacilli. It is not infrequent, for instance, to have several single positive cultures of tubercle bacilli obtained months or years apart with a large number of negative results in the interim. Radiologically, occasionally, the classical picture of tuberculosis superadded as it were, on silicotic nodules is seen; much more commonly however, this is not the case. Indeed, in the study already referred to, the percentage of silicotics with positive sputum, sometime, during the course of their disease was very similar in those with simple pneumoconiosis (small nodular shadows only) as in those with massive fibrosis (large conglomerate shadows usually in the upper parts of the lung fields).

2) ***Diabetes:*** It has been well documented that diabetics, particularly those with juvenile type diabetes are prone to develop tuberculosis. It has already been pointed out that tuberculous lesions in diabetes may occur in anterior parts of the lungs — this localization is most unusual in non-diabetics (Figure 5). In so far as tuberculosis is concerned, treatment is exactly the same, as it is in the non-diabetic individuals. The management of diabetes may present a problem as insulin requirements become greater, particularly in the initial stages of tuberculous disease and they sometimes seem to vary from day to day.

3) ***Chronic Alcoholism:*** Chronic alcoholism predisposes to tuberculosis. In a study on chronic alcoholic offenders(27) pulmonary tuberculosis was found to be an even more common disease than cirrhosis of the liver. The actual reason for this predisposition is not well known. Obviously, chronic alcoholics are more frequently exposed to infection due to their mode of life. Furthermore, there is often a coexistent under-nutrition due to neglect of normal diet.

Very little seems to be known about pathogenesis of pulmonary tuberculosis in alcoholics. Some of them seem to present with quite extensive disease, having had a normal chest x-ray only some months before. Whether these cases are a result of primary infection or indeed how common this particular sequence of events is, remains unknown. A serious study of the pathogenesis of pulmonary tuberculosis in alcoholics seems to be timely. The alcoholics respond and appear to tolerate antituberculous treatment as well as non-alcoholics; however it is often a difficult task to secure compliance with a full course of chemotherapy.

4) ***Pregnancy:*** It has been known for a long time that pregnancy effects tuberculosis adversely. In pre-antimicrobial days, women with active or even often those with inactive disease were cautioned against becoming pregnant. Tuberculosis was also one of the main medical indications for termination of pregnancy. It had been said that particularly dangerous are the first trimester of pregnancy and early puerperium. The latter danger had been attributed to the stress connected with the increased responsibilities in looking after a baby. The actual mechanism by which pregnancy activates tuberculosis is not known; it is almost certain that there is some connection between tuberculosis and "hormonal balance"; for instance, as has been pointed out

previously, post-primary pulmonary tuberculosis does not usually occur until puberty. So far as treatment is concerned, no real changes need to be made because of pregnancy. The teratogenic influence of Rifampin appears to be confined to laboratory animals given large doses of the drug. The possible damage to the eighth nerve of the unborn child when the mother is given Streptomycin has not been conclusively documented.

At the present time there are few contraindications to pregnancy as far as tuberculosis is concerned. Obviously, a woman with extensive disease and constitutional symptoms should be counselled not to become pregnant.

5) ***Under-nutrition:*** There is good evidence that under-nutrition and stress such as that seen during the war years may dramatically increase tuberculosis rates. This was well documented, for instance, in Holland during the Second World War(28). Although statistics are understandably lacking there is a strong hearsay evidence that tuberculosis was particularly rife in the concentration camps. There is also very good Norwegian data showing that underweight people develop tuberculosis more commonly than those of normal or excessive weight. Tuberculosis has always been a disease associated with poverty and poor socio-economic status. It is often difficult to disentangle individual factors responsible for the higher incidence of this disease among the poor; undoubtedly under-nutrition and frequent over-crowding with consequent ease of spread of infection are very important, although other factors such as emotional stress and lack of education with poor hygiene obviously often play a part.

6) ***Corticosteroids and immunosuppressive therapy:*** Every physician looking after tuberculosis cases sees some patients in whom the disease appears clearly related to corticosteroid therapy. The author sees several such cases every year. In the minds of most physicians there would seem to be no doubt that corticosteroids can reactivate established tuberculosis; the "healed" lesion in the lungs may reactivate and what is perhaps more significant miliary tuberculosis may develop. Corticosteroids are used widely in medical practice today but there has been no thorough study attempting to establish the actual risk of development of tuberculosis in patients treated with corticosteroids or other forms of immunosuppressive therapy. Such a

study is difficult as even if one could establish correctly the population of people treated with corticosteroids; the risk probably varies with the dosage used and with the duration of treatment. There are, of course, obvious host factors which surely will affect the risk, such as an individual with healed tuberculous lesions — an inactive case particularly one who has not received the benefit of adequate chemotherapy for the original disease. Also the disorder for which corticosteroids are given may influence the risk.

7) ***Gastrectomy:*** It is well documented that gastrectomy adds substantially to the risk of development of tuberculosis. The actual mechanism is unknown but it is probably related to consequent malnutrition. On the other hand, there are some suggestions that after gastrectomy as well as in some of the other predisposing conditions, there may be an impairment of cellular immunity, so important to tuberculosis.

8) ***Measles and Whooping Cough:*** Cases of miliary tuberculosis and of tuberculous meningitis in children in the past often appeared to originate at the time of an attack of measles or whooping cough. The actual mechanism is unknown. Possibly depression of cellular immunity co-exists with depression of tuberculin sensitivity in these individuals. Stress of general debilitating illness and possibly even severe cough may also all play a part.

CHAPTER IX

RELAPSES IN INACTIVE CASES, FIBROTIC LESIONS AND CHRONIC BACILLARY CASES

Individuals who have "recovered" from tuberculosis have a tendency to relapse. Such reactivations constitute somewhere between 10 and 15 percent of the total cases of active tuberculosis diagnosed in North America at the present time. Therefore, their contribution to the whole problem of tuberculosis is substantial. Risk of relapse is governed mainly by two factors:

1) The antimicrobial therapy given for the previous active episode of tuberculosis. In one of the studies in Canada(4) the average annual risk of reactivation (relapse) in patients with no chemotherapy (treated before chemotherapy era) was 0.7 percent, for those with poor chemotherapy the risk was 0.8 percent, while those with good chemotherapy (defined as treatment of longer duration than 12 months with at least two drugs, one of which was INH) was only 0.2 percent. The risk of relapse is, slightly greater in Eskimos and Indians than in white patients possibly due to the lower degree of natural resistance(3;4).

2) Time elapsing since recovery. In patients not treated with antimicrobials(29) the risk of reactivation is the greatest in the first few years following recovery and then diminishes substantially. The average annual risk in these patients was 4.4 percent in the first five years, 1.6 percent in the second 5 year period and dropped to 0.8 percent subsequently.

Curiously other factors, such as original extent of disease, previous bacillary status or previous surgery were found to be relatively less significant as far as risk of reactivation is concerned than the above two factors.

At present we still have some inactive cases "treated" prior to the antimicrobial era. These cases have a higher current risk of reactivation than those who received good chemotherapy just a year or two ago. With the passage of time the proportion of inactive cases who had adequate treatment will increase and therefore the overall risk of reactivation and its contribution to total active cases will diminish. This is understandable as most of the cases with "no treatment" and "poor treatment" had the active episode of their disease back in the 1930's, 1940's or early 1950's; they will gradually die out.

In patients whose disease has reactivated following previous antimicrobial treatment for active tuberculosis the pattern of resistance of tubercle bacilli is important as it does modify the treatment of a reactivated case. In our studies some 20 to 30 percent of patients who were previously treated harbour resistant tubercle bacilli(3,4) (Table 3). It must be realized however that this resistance pattern is intimately related both to the antimicrobial regimen prescribed initially and to the way patients take their drugs; the prevalence of secondary resistance may therefore vary quite widely.

TABLE 3

BACTERIAL RESISTANCE IN REACTIVATIONS OF TUBERCULOSIS PREVIOUSLY TREATED WITH ANTIMICROBIAL DRUGS

Total Number Previously Treated	Resistant Organisms		Susceptible	
	No.	%	No.	%
153	43	28.1	110	71.9

FIBROTIC LESIONS

Cases with fibrotic lesions are also known as those with "apical scarring" or as "presumed tuberculosis inactive." These are patients whose x-ray appearances are those of healed post-primary pulmonary tuberculosis, and who show a positive tuberculin reaction. They do not give any history of active disease, presumably they had it in the past, and "recovered" from it with no diagnosis and no treatment.

Such cases are frequently diagnosed on routine chest x-rays. Their risk of "reactivation" is fairly high, about 0.5 percent per annum. It must be remembered that the risk of reactivation, both in inactive cases and in fibrotic lesions is continuous; and after the first five years following active episodes it diminishes only very slightly in each succeeding year.

CHRONIC BACILLARY CASES OF TUBERCULOSIS

Chronic case is defined as one who is known to have tubercle bacilli in his sputum for more than two years. As will be discussed later, when the fate of a patient with pulmonary tuberculosis is considered, in the pre-antimicrobial era approximately one-third of cases of pulmonary tuberculosis became chronic — they were alive and excreted tubercle bacilli two years after diagnosis. When good chemotherapy is prescribed and taken the proportion of cases who become chronic is small (about 3 percent). It is, therefore, infrequent to see a chronic case in North America. On the other hand, in many developing countries the proportion of chronics among patients treated in "mass chemotherapy programs" may be as high as 25 percent. This is usually due to inadequate treatment regimens or to poor compliance with treatment. Chronic bacillary cases of tuberculosis are important when they constitute a significant part of the pool of infectors in the community. Unfortunately, to the author's knowledge there are no studies on chronic bacillary cases of pulmonary tuberculosis. We don't know how long they live, how they live — (the quality of life), the extent to which they are coming into contact with other people. They are however responsible for much of the primary resistance to drugs seen in the developing countries.

CHAPTER X

PROGNOSIS IN PULMONARY TUBERCULOSIS

Without chemotherapy the outlook for cases of pulmonary tuberculosis is quite grave though perhaps not as grave as is sometimes imagined. There has been a study in India(30) designed to answer the question of how tuberculosis behaves when there is no interference. Cases of tuberculosis were carefully diagnosed but no treatment was given. This study has furnished data on the fate of untreated bacteriologically positive cases. This data confirmed the observations made many years earlier in the pre-antimicrobial era in the western countries(31,32). Figure 6 taken from our study,(71) shows that after two years some 40 percent of such patients succumb to their disease, 30 percent become sputum negative (spontaneous cure) while another 30 percent are alive but remain sputum positive (chronic cases). After another three years a further 10 percent die; thus a 5 year survival was approximately 50 percent in this disease in the pre-antimicrobial era. The largely forgotten fact that one-third of patients with advanced disease with positive sputum smears recover on their own, should be kept in mind when claims are made that an inappropriate drug regimen cured a patient with bacterial resistance. It is impossible to assess the value of treatment of tuberculosis in the pre-antimicrobial era — to evaluate such measures as bed rest and collapse therapy; it is the author's feeling that while some patients were undoubtedly helped and their lives saved, these measures had probably little impact on the overall results.

Let us now look at the fate of cases treated with adequate chemotherapy. Data on this aspect (Figure 6) represent averages derived

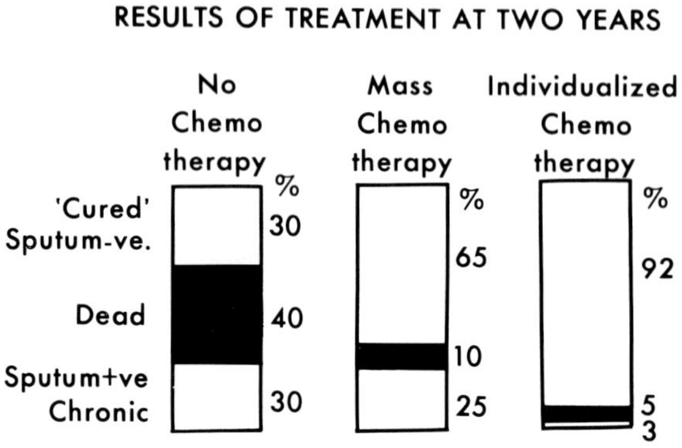

Figure 6. Results of treatment at two years.

from studies in England, Canada and Singapore(31). With such individual chemotherapy 92 percent of patients are cured, and 5 percent die. Most of these deaths are due to the very advanced stage of disease at the time diagnosis is reached. Only 3 percent of patients become chronic.

These findings may again be contrasted with what happens in the so-called "mass chemotherapy programs" in which standarized drug regimens are used. In some of those programs, some 65 percent of patients recover, 10 percent die but 25 percent remain chronic.

It is quite clear from these findings that it is relatively easy to prevent death from this disease. With no treatment, the patient has some 50 to 60 percent chance of surviving, and even "inappropriate" chemotherapy (e.g., INH alone) will save a lot of lives. The price for such treatment is, however, creation of chronic patients with INH resistant bacilli and eventually increase in primary resistance to INH in the community.

CHAPTER XI

TREATMENT OF TUBERCULOSIS

It is perhaps true to say that prior to the antimicrobial era, there was no effective treatment of tuberculosis. In management of a tuberculosis patient we went through the stage of exercise such as horse riding (whoever collapses first, horse or the patient), followed by the era of general rest reaching its extreme in absolute bedrest in a sanatorium when the patient was hardly allowed to move for months on end. Then came an era of securing "localized rest" for the affected lung or lungs by measures such as artificial pneumothorax, pneumoperitoneum (usually combined with a phrenic nerve crush), or by a thoracoplasty.

Resection of the diseased portion of the lung was too dangerous before antimicrobial coverage became available. It came into vogue in the early years of the antimicrobial era, only to be found unnecessary a short time later.

Sanatoria were being built, often in beautiful surroundings of pine woods or in the mountains and patients with tuberculosis confined to such institutions stayed there frequently for periods of years. Whatever the value of the sanatorium treatment was to individual patients, it had, undoubtedly, performed a most useful function by the removal of a large number of sources of infection from the community. In many developed countries, there was a great expansion of the building programs of the sanatoria and tuberculosis hospitals after the Second World War as the demand for the beds was great and the waiting lists quite lengthy. In many areas, this demand was only met by the late 1940's or early 1950's just at the time of the introduction of antimicrobial treatment. This created almost immediately a headache for administrators — what to do with the empty beds.

There were short periods earlier in this century when measures thought to be more specific enjoyed shortlived popularity, such as treatment with tuberculin, calcium or gold injections etc. There was even a large international congress on treatment of tuberculosis with radiotherapy.

How much good all of those measures achieved is impossible to assess. As has already been pointed out, about one third of patients with advanced disease with positive sputum smears recover without any help. Probably this proportion is somewhat larger in less advanced cases. It seems reasonable to expect that rest, both general and local (collapse therapy) together with good nutrition may have increased to a limited degree this recovery rate simply by enhancing the tendency of tuberculosis to heal and by increasing natural resistance to tubercle bacilli.

TREATMENT TODAY

Hospitalization: In the developed countries, there is usually no difficulty in finding a bed for a tuberculous patient and for providing him with a period of hospitalization with little or no cost to himself.

What are the aims of hospitalization? The first one is isolation — preventing the patient from infecting others around him. Tuberculosis is not a very infectious disease and for practical purposes only patients with positive sputum smears infect some of their contacts. They usually do so before the diagnosis is established as subsequently their personal hygiene improves with the understanding of how tuberculosis is spread; furthermore, the antimicrobial treatment very soon renders them much less infectious, and eventually, non-infectious. However, in some patients such as some chronic alcoholics, these measures may not be accepted by the patient. In such cases isolation in hospital may be essential.

Patients who are very ill, with marked constitutional symptoms — high fever and those with hemoptysis — also require initial hospitalization. Not infrequently there are reasonable social indications for hospitalization; tuberculosis is often the disease of the poor and if poverty is extreme it would be inhuman to leave the patient in his environment when other facilities are readily available.

Establishment of an appropriate drug regimen was, in the past, considered to be an indication for hospitalization. This with standardized, relatively non-toxic drug regimens, is no longer really applicable. There is, of course, a place for hospitalization of a patient who started treatment on an out-patient basis but who developed serious side effects or simply cannot tolerate the drugs. A frequent reason given for hospitalization or for keeping a patient in for an unduly long period is that he will stop taking his medications or will take them irregularly once discharged. This is of course, not an indication for prolonged hospital treatment, but is an indictment of authorities for not providing sufficient facilities for supervised chemotherapy in the community.

In a recent study(33) one of the author's associates compared knowledge of tuberculosis in patients who were initially hospitalized for their disease, in those who were started as out-patients and in controls who never had tuberculosis. This study showed that while all the patients with tuberculosis have very poor knowledge of their disease, those initially hospitalized knew appreciably more than those treated as outpatients from the beginning. Obviously, it would be foolish to hospitalize a patient simply to teach him about tuberculosis. What is needed is a much greater effort and emphasis on the patient's education whether in the hospital or on the outside. For those treated as outpatients from the start adequate teaching is often lacking.

The above discussion related to developed countries with relative abundance of beds for tuberculous patients. In developing countries it would be foolish to commit financial resources to establishment of new tuberculous institutions; indeed it has been shown in Madras, India that hospitalization has no effect on incidence of tuberculosis among close contacts.

ANTIMICROBIAL DRUGS

Although antimicrobial agents now at our disposal are very effective and have changed substantially the whole picture of tuberculosis, it does not seem unlikely that new, even more powerful drugs will be developed in the future. It is to be regretted, in view of the still existing tremendous problem of tuberculosis in the world, that the pharmaceutical industry does not apparently place a high priority on the development of new anti-tuberculous agents.

Not so long ago it was customary to divide antimicrobial drugs into two or three groups: those called first line, second line and third line drugs. First line drugs, Isoniazid, Streptomycin and PAS (later replaced by Ethambutol), were considered standard chemotherapy given to all the newly diagnosed cases with sensitive tubercle bacilli for periods up to 24 months. Second and third line drugs were reserved for re-treatment cases and for those who for one reason or another could not tolerate some of the first line drugs. Thanks to the research in the area of antimicrobial treatment, in which the Medical Research Council of Great Britain assumed the leading and most important role, there has been in recent years, considerable development of new effective short-course regimens. This made the division of antimicrobial agents into first and second line etc. largely meaningless.

In Table 4 these drugs are divided into most effective (with bacteriocidal action) and those less effective with mainly bacteriostatic effect.

TABLE 4

ANTIMICROBIAL AGENTS IN TUBERCULOSIS

Drug	Method of Administration	Usual Daily Dose	Frequency
Most Effective			
INH	Oral—tablet	300 mg (5 mg/kilo)	Once daily
Rifampin	Oral—capsule	450-600 mg	Once daily—fasting
Streptomycin	IM	0.75-1.0 g	Once daily
Pyrazinamide	Oral—tablet	40 mg/kilo (max—3 gm daily)	Once daily
Less Effective			
Ethambutol	Oral—tablet	15 mg/kg	Once daily
Ethionamide	Oral—tablet Rectal—supp.	1 g	Two equal doses
Capreomycin	IM	1 g (max 20 mg/kilo)	Once daily
Cycloserine	Oral	500-750 mg	Two or three equal doses
PAS	Oral—tablet liquid, granules	12-15 g	Once daily
Thiacetazone	Oral—tablet	150 mg	Once daily

TREATMENT REGIMENS

There has been an almost revolutionary progress in chemotherapy in the last few years and it is likely that this progress will continue. Established long-term courses of treatment relying mainly on INH, Streptomycin and PAS (or Ethambutol) have recently been replaced by short-course chemotherapy(73) relying chiefly on the two main bacteriocidal drugs, Isoniazid and Rifampin given together. It is not unlikely that whatever is written here today will be replaced in the near future by new and better regimens.

The aim of antimicrobial treatment at least in developed countries is to cure the patient completely so that there is no, or only a very small chance of relapse. This aim may, for economic reasons, be somewhat modified in developing countries: in those countries the aim could justifiably be to cure over 90 percent of patients in the most effective, but also in the most economical way, and to accept a small chance of relapse, provided that it can be dealt with satisfactorily by further treatment. Of course, both points of view are right and are optimal for the wealthy and for the poorer countries.

Modern Chemotherapy: In the present state of our knowledge tuberculosis should be treated with the two most powerful drugs—Isoniazid and Rifampin. Provided that tubercle bacilli are sensitive to both drugs, treatment should continue for nine months, if our aim is to effect complete cure with no significant chance of relapse. As such chemotherapy is expensive due to the high cost of Rifampin, the total duration of treatment may be reduced to six months; it is then necessary to follow patients to discover the few who will relapse. The tubercle bacilli in these relapses are almost invariably drug sensitive and can be given a second course of the same chemotherapy. As at the beginning of treatment we very seldom have information relating to drug sensitivity of the tubercle bacilli, a third drug should be added (usually Ethambutol) and continued until the results of drug sensitivity are available.

It has been customary to divide treatment into the initial intensive phase, followed by a somewhat less intensive continuation phase. In regimens containing Isoniazid and Rifampin with disease caused by sensitive organisms such a division may possibly prove unnecessary in the future. It is advantageous in many patients to utilize two to three times a week regimens consisting of high dose of INH (15 mgm /kgm body weight) and an "ordinary" 600 mg dose of Rifampin under complete supervision. This is mandatory in patients such as chronic alcoholics who appear "a priori" to be likely not to comply with treatment; however, many seemingly cooperative individuals also fail to take their drugs regularly and would benefit from supervision. Intermittent regimen is also less expensive(34).

In a few patients whose attitude to disease and often to life in general is such that they appear unlikely to comply with any regimen of treatment and who are therefore hospitalized, the author uses regimens consisting of Isoniazid, Rifampin, Pyrazinamide and Streptomycin. This is thought to be the most powerful regimen available and hopefully an appreciable proportion of these patients will be cured even if the total duration of treatment is only three or four months.

ANTIMICROBIAL DRUGS (ADVERSE REACTIONS)

These are usually divided into local (e.g., local inflammatory reaction following Streptomycin injection or gastritis due to PAS), hypersensitivity (e.g. skin rashes, fever) and toxic (e.g., vestibular damage due to Streptomycin). The actual mechanism of some reactions e.g., hepatitis occurring during Isoniazid or Rifampin treatment is still not firmly established.

Isoniazid

The most serious side effect of Isoniazid is the development of hepatitis. The customary dose for adults is 300 mgm per day but at least one country uses 200 mgm while a number use 400 mgm as a routine. Hepatitis is perhaps more frequently seen in chemoprophylaxis when INH is given alone, than in treatment when Isoniazid is given with other drugs. Some authorities believe however that Rifampin facilitates the development of INH hepatitis.

Incidence of probable INH induced hepatitis is related to age; it is very seldom seen in children; it is then reported to rise progressively with age, being 0.3 percent in persons between 20–34; 1.2 percent in those between 35–49; and 2.3 percent in those between 50–64 years of age(35). Because of the danger of hepatitis, monitoring of abnormalities of liver function is often undertaken.

Elevation of SGOT (serum glutamic oxaloacetic transaminase) to a minor degree is common, occurring in some ten percent of individuals receiving INH. Similar findings are also often seen after abuse of alcohol and the reason for an abnormal result in an alcoholic patient is often difficult to ascertain. It is not necessary to interrupt treatment because of this biochemical abnormality but tests should be repeated and the patient watched more carefully.

Peripheral neuropathy due to deficiency of pyridoxine (Vitamin B6) is very uncommon in developed countries where nutrition is adequate; consequently the use of small prophylactic doses of Pyridoxine in routine treatment is unnecessary. In some patients with previous psychotic episodes Isoniazid may precipitate another episode but this is uncommon. Aplastic anemia, lupus erythematosus and polyarthritis have all been described but are exceedingly rare. As with any other medication, frequently there are effects which are likely imaginary. One of the author's patients was convinced that Isoniazid stopped him from getting colds from which he suffered a lot previous to his treatment. An elderly silicotic complained to the Compensation Board that Isoniazid — chemoprophylaxis given to him by the author, caused impotence. It was pleasing to be able to counter by a statement from two, even older, silicotics that "they never had it so good" and would like to stay on the drug for the rest of their lives.

Rifampin

Perhaps the greatest disadvantage of Rifampin is its high cost, which precludes many patients in poorer countries from receiving this drug.

There is still some discussion whether Rifampin is hepatotoxic by itself or whether it somehow facilitates the liver toxicity induced by Isoniazid. It must be emphasized however that hepatitis is uncommon on regimens containing Rifampin and Isoniazid.

When Rifampin is taken intermittently either by design, in intermittent supervised regimens, or because of forgetfulness of the patient, peculiar sensitivity reactions occasionally occur. These include fever, shortness of breath, cough, skin rash, abdominal pain, and very occasionally thrombocytopoenic purpura. In intermittent regimens these reactions occur more commonly when Rifampin is given once a week than when it is given twice a week. When the drugs are taken three times a week, these reactions virtually never occur.

There is evidence that Rifampin is an immunosuppressant; the practical significance of this is not apparent. There were also teratogenic effects when very large doses of Rifampin were fed to pregnant rats; however many pregnant women have received treatment with Rifampin with no apparent increase in fetal abnormalities and it seems unlikely that the drug is dangerous when taken during pregnancy. Rifampin also interferes with the contraceptive pill, and a variety of other drugs.

Because of its wide bacterial spectrum, Rifampin is also increasingly used in the treatment of other infections in combination with other antimicrobial agents; this raises the possibility of incidental increase of resistance of tubercle bacilli to this valuable drug.

Streptomycin

Streptomycin was the first of the antituberculous drugs; it was discovered by Waksman in 1947. It is still a valuable drug although its bacteriocidal activity is less than that of either Isoniazid or Rifampin.

Hypersensitivity reactions with fever and skin rash are common; they tend to occur a few weeks (usually 3-4) after commencement of treatment. Occasionally, fever is the only manifestation of hypersensitivity and the clinician is worried about other possible causes of fever such as exacerbation of the tuberculous process or a superadded infection. One of the clues suggesting that fever is a manifestation of hypersensitivity to Streptomycin is that in spite of high temperature the patient does not appear very ill. The time of occurrence, a few weeks after commencement of treatment and the presence of eosinophilia are also helpful.

Occasionally, patients complain of circumoral paresthesia and of feeling "fuzzy" a few hours after receiving Streptomycin; the cause may be some impurity as the reaction often disappears when another preparation of Streptomycin is used. The most important side effects of Streptomycin are toxic — related to dosage. Streptomycin damages the vestibular part of the eighth nerve. In the 1950's, it used to be said that when a waiter spilled soup on your trousers, the likely diagnosis was tuberculosis. In order to avoid vestibular damage, the patient who is receiving full doses of daily Streptomycin should be watched and asked about dizziness. This subjective symptom comes sometime before any objective signs of vestibular damage, and it is wise to discontinue Streptomycin at such a time or at least to diminish the dose in a substantial way. As Streptomycin is excreted by kidney, vestibular damage occurs much quicker in patients with renal impairment. This is why such investigations as urinalysis, BUN and creatinine should always be done before deciding on the dose of Streptomycin. It is customary to use one gram daily in people under the age of 45 or 50 and to use .75 grams in older individuals.

Pyrazinamide

This is a very important antimicrobial agent and is now used much more frequently together with other antimicrobial drugs in routine treatment of newly diagnosed cases. In the past it was considered a second line drug to be used only in retreatment. At the time, it acquired a reputation of being very toxic, a reputation which it does not quite deserve. It is true that side effects of pyrazinamide are not uncommon and are occasionally serious. Nevertheless, the vast majority of patients can take this drug without any difficulty. The main side effects relate to hepatotoxicity which is occasionally serious, unless the drug is promptly withdrawn. Elevation of uric acid probably occurs in every patient taking pyrazinamide; curiously even with quite high levels of uric acid, gout is uncommon. Arthialgia apparently unrelated to hyperuricaemia is not infrequent.

Ethambutol

This is a commonly used drug which has replaced the more toxic and a more cumbersome to take PAS. It is a weak drug and there are several studies suggesting that the combination of INH and PAS is slightly more potent than that of INH and Ethambutol. Ethambutol should be used merely as a "resistance-preventing drug" added to the combination of Isoniazid and Rifampin. The rationale for using Ethambutol is obviously the somewhat unlikely possibility in a caucasian patient that bacilli are INH resistant and therefore to give him Isoniazid and Rifampin only, would be tantamount to treatment with Rifampin alone. By the time the INH resistance is reported, the organisms would almost inevitably have developed Rifampin resistance. When the sensitivity report comes back and shows no resistance to either Isoniazid or Rifampin, Ethambutol can and should be discontinued as it adds little to the potency of treatment but does add slightly to toxicity.

The major toxic effect of Ethambutol is optic neuritis. This is dose-related and is very infrequent, when the low dose of 15 mg/kg is used. It was more frequent in the past when the higher 25 mg/kg of body weight dose was used. It is customary to test the vision of patients on Ethambutol every few weeks. The author is somewhat unconvinced that such routine testing is of real benefit to the patients. As with all other anti-tuberculous drugs, it is essential to educate the patient about the nature of possible side effects, as symptoms usually antedate abnormal tests. Undoubtedly, however, monitoring of this kind protects the physician in case of possible litigation.

Other antituberculous agents

It is unnecessary to discuss at any length other drugs as they are used quite infrequently in practice.

PAS is still occasionally used particularly in children as a companion drug to Isoniazid. The advantage of such a regimen is doubtful as children can take readily the more potent antimicrobial agents. The common side effect of PAS is gastric irritation with consequent dyspepsia, abdominal pain and occasional diarrhea. Hypersensitivity reactions are common.

Cycloserine is a neurotoxic drug and in effective dosage (one gram a day), it occasionally causes seizures. It is the only antituberculous agent which has to be given in divided doses, e.g., 250 mg qid. All other drugs can safely be taken once a day usually on an empty stomach, as this secures absorption of Rifampin.

Ethionomide is a potent gastric irritant, and because of that it is often given twice daily or as a suppository; in addition it is hepatotoxic.

Capreomycin has similar side effects to Streptomycin.

CHAPTER XII

TUBERCULIN TEST

Tuberculin was initially discovered by Robert Koch at the turn of the century as an extract from the supernatant of the culture of the tubercle bacilli. This substance known as "OLD TUBERCULIN" is still occasionally used. Siebert working in the United States in the 1930's produced a much more refined tuberculin, PPD Tuberculin (purified protein derivative). The large batch of PPD produced by Siebert designated as PPD-S became a recognized international standard with which other tuberculins, produced in many countries, are supposed to be compared.

Tuberculin surveys early in this century revealed that in cities of Europe most children were positive reactors by the age of 15. Therefore, until the 1940's it was assumed that there was little point in tuberculin testing any adult as the result is bound to be positive. It was also believed that tuberculin reaction is a specific reaction indicating only infection with tubercle bacilli and that this reaction is persistent — "once positive always positive." It has also been known that individuals vaccinated with BCG (Bacillus Calmette-Guerin) also show a positive tuberculin reaction.

The next chapter in the story of our understanding of tuberculin reaction begins with the studies conducted by the Tuberculosis Research Office established in Copenhagen after the Second World War under the direction of Dr. Caroll Palmer. Carefully trained testing teams were sent to different areas of the world and measured accurately the diameter of tuberculin reactions. The results of these studies have proven to be most interesting. Tuberculin reactions due to infection with tubercle bacilli were shown to be relatively large with the mean diameter between 15 and 20 mm of induration and a pattern following the normal distribution curve. In many areas, particularly the low-lying areas of the tropics, there was, in addition, a very large number of small reactions superimposed, as it were, on the left limb of this normal distribution curve. The workers at the Tuberculosis Research office have postulated that there must be another source of sensitivity distinct from infection with tubercle bacilli accounting for this "low-grade" sensitivity. Some years later, Palmer and his co-workers (now working in the U.S. Public Health Service) have proven conclusively that these small reactions are caused by infections with non-tuberculous mycobacteria the so-called atypical mycobacteria(36). At about the same time, and surprisingly apparently independently, a child-oriented program of tuberculosis control was introduced in the U.S.(37). The basis of this program was to test and periodically retest the school children. It was thought, that positive reactors and particularly recent convertors (those whose reactions have changed from negative to positive) would readily lead public health authorities to sources of infection. The main reason for the failure of this program lay in the fact that undue reliance had been placed on the specificity of the tuberculin reaction.

"Atypical" mycobacterial infections are a frequent cause of "non-specific" tuberculin sensitivity, even in temperate climates like that of British Columbia(38). The tuberculin reactions or rather cross-reactions caused by these infections tend to be small, under 10 mm in diameter, but are occasionally larger (up to 20 mm) when an ordinary 5 TU dose of tuberculin is used (Table 5). With a larger dose of Tuberculin (e.g., 250 TU) most of the individuals infected with atypical

TABLE 5

RESULTS OF TESTING HIGH SCHOOL AND UNIVERSITY STUDENTS WITH TUBERCULIN (PPD-S) AND ATYPICAL ANTIGEN—(PPD-GAUSE) BRITISH COLUMBIA 1965–1969

Number Tested	TBN Reaction Greater		Atypical Reaction Greater		Reactions Equal	
	No.	%	No.	%	No.	%
2884	109	3.8	538	18.6	13	0.5

mycobacteria show cross-reactivity. The prevalence of "atypical" mycobacterial infections varies from area to area even to a greater extent than that of tuberculous infection. In low-lying tropical areas, these infections are extremely common and probably everybody is infected in their childhood(39). In more temperate areas, like British Columbia, Canada, where the author conducted his studies the prevalence of these infections is lower, but in children it is still appreciably greater than that of tuberculous infection. The evidence which is available indicates that atypical infections do not occur in cold climates, for instance in Alaska(40). Thus, tuberculin reactions to an ordinary 5 TU dose of tuberculin (for example those of 12 mm in diameter) will have different significance in children in Florida, children in British Columbia or children in Alaska. These differences are also applicable to different age groups. This is due to the fact that the risk of tuberculous infection has been declining very rapidly; therefore in older age groups a larger proportion of small reactions are due to infections with tubercle bacilli than in the younger group.

The distinction between specific tuberculous infection and atypical mycobacterial infections can be fairly reliably established by simultaneous testing of the individual with tuberculin (PPD-S) and with antigens prepared from "atypical" mycobacteria. The rationale for such testing lies both in experimental and in epidemiological work showing that the reaction is always larger to the homogenous antigen (i.e., one prepared from the same mycobacterium with which the animal has been infected) than that obtained with heterogenous ones(41). In the author's experience the best antigens for atypical infections are those prepared by the Centre for Disease Control, in Atlanta, Georgia, particularly PPD-G (Gause) and PPD-B (Battey).

When these antigens are given to patients with bacteriologically proven tuberculosis, practically always the reaction to tuberculin is larger than that elicited by PPD-G and PPD-B(38). Simultaneous testing of a school population in British Columbia reveals large numbers of students in whom the reaction to PPD-G is the largest, to PPD-B usually slightly smaller, while the reaction to PPD-S is much smaller or absent. A small proportion of students however react in exactly the same way as tuberculous patients, with reaction to PPD-S being the largest. Individuals showing larger reactions to atypical mycobacterial antigens than to tuberculin have almost certainly been infected with atypical mycobacteria: it is, however, impossible to be sure which particular mycobacterium was responsible for the infection. Individuals in whom the largest reaction is to tuberculin (PPD-S) have very likely been infected with tubercle bacilli.

It must be emphasized that in the majority of individuals infected with atypical mycobacteria as evidenced by reactions to "atypical" antigens, there is no cross-reactivity to the usual 5 TU dose of tuberculin, although practically all react when a large (250 TU) dose of PPD is used.

BCG vaccination induces a degree of tuberculin sensitivity which is similar, though usually slightly stronger, than that due to atypical mycobacterial infections. The actual size of tuberculin reactions following a BCG vaccination varies greatly depending on the particular vaccine used. With the Connaught vaccine used in student nurses by us, the average reaction to 5 TU PPD-S is 17.8 mm with 10 percent of student nurses showing no reaction whatsoever (0 mm). When these BCG vaccinated non-reactors are tested with 250 TU, practically all of them react. Tuberculin sensitivity due to BGC vaccination tends to wane quite quickly unless repeated tuberculin tests act as a "booster."

Waning of tuberculin reactivity is a well described, though perhaps an insufficiently studied phenomenon(42). At the time of tuberculin conversion following primary tuberculous infection, the degree of sensitivity is very high: the reactions can be elicited with very small doses of tuberculin(43) or if standard (5 TU dose) is used, large reactions are common. The high degree of hypersensitivity diminishes fairly rapidly over a period of months and in some it may wane to below the level arbitrarily chosen as the lower limit of a positive reaction after a period of years. Such small reactions can be "boosted" by repeated tuberculin tests, by infection with "atypical' mycobacteria, by BCG vaccination or reinfection with tubercle bacilli. If a previously infected individual, whose tuberculin test is negative, is retested with the same (5 TU) dose of tuberculin the test frequently becomes positive. However, an individual who has never encountered any mycobacterial infection cannot be rendered tuberculin positive by repeated injections of tuberculin.

Tuberculin sensitivity can also be temporarily depressed by a large number of factors; among the best known is severe constitutional illness such as that seen in patients with advanced tuberculosis; by viral infections including vaccinations with live viruses, by cortico-steroids and, allegedly, also contraceptive pills.

It is obvious from the above discussion that tuberculin sensitivity is a complex phenomenon and that we have probably placed too heavy demands on this simple test in tuberculosis control programs, particularly in those which are based on repeated testing. Tuberculin conversion must not be equated with the primary tuberculosis infection, although of course all primary infections are accompanied by conversion. It is likely that in North America the majority of conversions are due to the boosting of pre-existing sensitivity whether specific or non-specific. Some conversions may also be due to new atypical mycobacterial infections and others to the fact that a previous supposedly negative reaction was for instance the result of intercurrent viral infection. However, if a definite conversion occurs in a contact of an active case of tuberculosis obviously the probability of true tuberculous infection is very high.

Methods of testing: Intradermal test (Mantoux test) in which a small amount, (0.1 ml) of tuberculin dilution usually 5 TU PPD-S equivalent is injected into the epidermis is the most reliable method of testing. The uncertainties regarding tuberculin sensitivity discussed above are obviously greatly magnified when various percutaneous methods (Tine test, Heaf test or Scratch test) are used: in these tests a large dose of tuberculin is applied through punctures in the epidermis, and therefore false positive and false negative reactions are common. Use of the Heaf test with few false negative reactions could be justified, provided that positive reaction is always followed by the Manotoux test. Unfortunately, false negative reactions occur commonly with Tine and Scratch tests rendering them of little value.

Although the technique of the Mantoux test is relatively easy, it is essential that it be very meticulous; for research purposes personnel must be trained thoroughly in the technique of testing and reading. Exactly the right amount (0.1 ml) has to be injected into the superficial layers of the epidermis. Although the volar side of the forearm is traditionally used, there are advantages to using the dorsal side of the forearm as the resulting induration seems to be easier to measure accurately. The reaction is read some 48 to 72 hours later and the transverse diameter of the induration should be carefully measured and recorded. It is, incidentally, quite easy to spot an inexperienced reader in tuberculin survey, as he will show a tendency to call the reactions 5, 10, 15, 20 mm etc., whereas an experienced reader will have a pretty even distribution of recorded reactions by millimeter.

No two batches of tuberculin are exactly the same even if they are prepared by the same manufacturer. Before careful standardization of tuberculin became mandatory there were very substantial differences between various tuberculins as we have shown in a study on patients with previously documented active tuberculosis who received Mantoux tests with four tuberculins allegedly of similar strength(22). The strongest of the four tuberculin gave an average reaction of 21.5 mm, and 3 percent of patients showed no reactions (0 mm) while with the weakest the average reaction was 5.6 mm with 23 percent nonreactors. Nowadays, new batches of PPD are carefully compared with PPD-S in those infected with tubercle bacilli. However different preparations differ in the degree of cross reactivity in individuals infected with atypical mycobacteria. Thus, even when a new batch of tuberculin causes reactions which are exactly the same as those elicited by PPD-S in tuberculous patients, the size of reactions may differ when these two preparations are used in individuals infected with atypical mycobacteria. PPD-S has been for instance shown to be a "more specific" antigen than RT 23, a tuberculin used very widely in many developing countries(44).

The recommended dose of tuberculin in North America is 5 TU of PPD-S "equivalent." This is because, most studies on tuberculin sensitivity have been conducted with 5 TU PPD-S which had no addition of a stabilizer (such as Tween-80). In such solutions, there is rapid adsorption of tuberculin onto the glass of the vial and after a week or so the actual strength of tuberculin remaining in the solution is somewhere about 2 TU. In order to assure comparability of various PPD products in North America, the new products containing Tween-80 are compared with "aged" PPD-S (without Tween-80) and designated as bio-equivalent to 5 TU PPD-S. This actually compares also reasonably well with 2 TU of RT 23 used in many countries of the world.

What constitutes a positive tuberculin reaction? The above discussion should have made it clear that there cannot be any strict scientific dividing lines between the positive, "doubtful" and negative reactions. The American Thoracic Society after a great deal of consideration decided to place the lowest limit of positive reaction at 10 mm(45); this appeared to be the most reasonable compromise, taking into account the findings of tuberculin testing studies in children in various areas of the country. Most of the reactions in most areas of the U.S. which were below 10 mm were likely caused by atypical mycobacteria, while most of those over 10 mm were likely due to tuberculous infection. However this arbitrary diameter of 10 mm to 5 TU PPD-S is often inadequate when one suspects tuberculosis in middle age or elderly individuals. Such a patient may have tuberculosis even when his reaction fails to meet the 10 mm standard. Similarly, in contacts of tuberculosis cases, the probability is that smaller reactions are due to tuberculous infection and the American Thoracic Society recommended that all reactions above 5 mm be considered positive in this group. Size of tuberculin reaction as well as that elicited by atypical antigens is related to age. Generally, children have smaller reactions than adults and young children show the smallest reactions(46).

In recent years, many attempts have been made to produce a specific tuberculin which would not give any cross reactions. This would obviously solve many current problems with tuberculin testing; however, these attempts have not yet met with any success.

In conclusion, it may be said that the tuberculin test is a useful auxiliary tool in clinical diagnosis and in epidemiological studies in tuberculosis. Most of the patients with tuberculosis show a positive reaction to 5 TU of PPD. All individuals not infected with tubercle bacilli or any other mycobacteria show a completely negative result even when a large dose of tuberculin is used. Tuberculin reaction should, however, always be interpreted within the particular clinical or epidemiological context and one should avoid being dogmatic. When the reaction is negative, the individual probably was not infected with tubercle bacilli. When it is positive, the individual was infected with mycobacteria which might have been tubercle bacilli or atypical mycobacteria or he was vaccinated with BCG. Generally, it is unwise to make important decisions such as starting a course of chemoprophylaxis on the basis of a tuberculin reaction alone, without taking into account such factors as the size of the reaction, contact history, results of previous testing etc.

Finally, one often meets with the belief that large tuberculin reactions signify a dangerous clinical situation, increasing greatly the likelihood of tuberculous disease. Large reactions are associated with a slightly higher risk of development of tuberculosis than the smaller ones for two reasons. Firstly, persons with smaller reactions contain a larger proportion of individuals with non-specific tuberculin sensitivity, showing no risk of tuberculous disease; secondly larger reactions tend to occur early following a recent infection and consequently carry the additional risk of early morbidity. One should remember, however, that the vast majority of individuals with large tuberculin reactions do not have, and will not develop, tuberculosis.

CHAPTER XIII

CHEST X-RAY

Radiologic examination of the chest is a time honoured method used in the diagnosis of pulmonary tuberculosis. The chest x-ray is, of course, a very good diagnostic tool but we know now that we have made a mistake in the past by according to it an overwhelming importance. When tuberculosis was a common disease in western countries, any shadow that looked like tuberculosis was likely due to this disease. With the decline of tuberculosis rates, this is no longer true. The International Union Against Tuberculosis conducted an interesting study in which twenty expert readers from several countries read the same 205 chest x-ray films(47). The degree of variation in interpretation between these expert readers was astonishing. The main difference related to etiology (tuberculous and non-tuberculous) and to clinical status (active or inactive disease). In that study, 29 percent of non-tuberculous conditions (in tuberculin negative persons) were wrongly diagnosed as active tuberculosis. On the other hand 13 percent of sputum positive cases were not diagnosed as tuberculosis. It is obvious, therefore, that even internationally recognized experts disagree which lesions are and which are not tuberculous. Furthermore, if tuberculous, it is often also difficult to be sure from radiological appearance whether we are dealing with an active process requiring treatment or with inactive disease.

The radiologic examination is also traditionally used to gauge the progress of active disease under treatment. Even today in numerous sanatoria and tuberculosis hospitals the focal point at staff conferences is an illuminated x-ray viewing box and experts study the changing radiological picture in great detail. Indeed, in most cases of active tuberculosis, the radiological picture changes quite dramatically under the influence of antimicrobial therapy. The cavities usually become smaller and then close. "Fresh" infiltrates tend to become smaller and sometimes disappear completely. At other times, particularly when one is dealing with considerable fibrotic component in the lesions, the radiological appearances change very little although the patient is being cured from his disease. While not decrying the value of radiology in following the course of disease, it must be emphasized that careful perusal of the bacteriological chart on which the results of periodic examination of the sputum are recorded gives much more important insight into the progress of the disease.

CHAPTER XIV

BACTERIOLOGY

While it has been realized since the turn of the century that bacteriology constitutes a very important tool in diagnosis, its importance seemed to have been somewhat submerged by the prominence given to chest x-rays since the 1930's. The stimulus of the research in India which gave bacteriology new prominence, arose primarily from the search for the cheapest and most reliable diagnostic methods capable of bringing to light large numbers of cases who had limited access to traditional medical facilities. Microscopic examination of the sputum for acid fast bacilli in patients with chronic productive cough was found to be an excellent method of diagnosis of large numbers of such cases.

Another important fact emphasizing the overwhelming value of bacteriological examination was the introduction of antimicrobial treatment of tuberculosis in the 1950's. Both in the chemotherapy trials and in following the course of disease in individual patients, conversion of sputum from positive to negative was found to be the most reliable objective method of judging the effectiveness of treatment.

As was discussed previously, positive sputum smears usually indicate fairly advanced disease; it has been stated that a minimum of 100,000 tubercle bacilli per millilitre of sputum are necessary to be seen on microscopy. It is, of course, essential to obtain a proper specimen of sputum (not saliva) and to select suitable material from the specimen — particles and pus.

Sputum culture, although technically not difficult, requires a prolonged time of 4 to 10 weeks of growth on suitable media (solidified agar media are generally used in North America). Apparently only a few hundred bacilli per ml of sputum are sufficient to be detected by culture(48).

Animal innoculation has largely been abandoned; it has about the same sensitivity as culture of the bacilli.

Bacteriological examination of the sputum can, of course, be used as a primary case finding measure even in the Western countries. It is particularly indicated in geographically remote areas where x-ray facilities are located a long distance away. It is also indicated when the patient with suggestive symptoms is suspected to be unreliable (e.g., some chronic alcoholics); it is preferable to give such a patient a sputum container and ask him to cough up some phlegm there and then, than giving him an x-ray requisition to the neighbouring clinic or radiology department to which he may never report. It is also preferable to x-rays in situations where radiology is difficult, e.g., old people's homes.

When one suspects tuberculosis because of suggestive symptoms, or because of radiological abnormality it is customary to give three sputum containers and to ask the patient to expectorate into them on three successive mornings. Occasionally, twenty-four hour specimens are better. Some cases, with low bacterial population or scanty sputum will, of course, show a positive bacteriological results only when a larger number of specimens than three are submitted. It was shown in one of the studies in India that when one specimen of sputum is collected for culture the prevalence of disease has to be multiplied by 1.67 in order to obtain prevalence resulting from examination of multiple specimens(49).

There are several methods of quantitating the number of bacilli seen in the sputum smears. Among them the earliest and the one that is still frequently used was designed by Gaffky; the findings are expressed as Gaffky count rated from 1 to 10. The response to treatment may be monitored fairly accurately by repeat count of the bacilli in the sputum. If the count does not diminish over a matter of weeks, or if there is "a fall and rise phenomenon," then the probability is that the bacilli are resistant to the drugs used or that the patient is not taking the medication.

SPUTUM CONVERSION

The rapidity of sputum conversion with modern chemotherapy is, of course, an indication of the effectiveness of treatment. There is evidence that even in advanced cases with positive smears, a relatively short period of treatment renders them less infectious(50). Nevertheless, bacteriological conversion of sputum is a cardinal sign of response to treatment. Some years ago, we were trying to compare the speed of sputum conversion in the Eskimo patients with the white patients(51). We have concluded that there was no difference between the two races, but we have incidentally accumulated some data on the speed of bacteriological conversion. These cases were treated with two or three drugs including INH but not including Rifampin. We have found that in cases who are initially smear positive it takes approximately six weeks for conversion of smears and another month for culture conversion. Patients who are originally smear negative take a little less than a month for conversion of the cultures to negative. The speed of conversion in individual patients varies considerably with the extent of disease; the minimal cases converting twice as fast as those with far advanced disease.

When Rifampin is added to the drug regimen containing INH (provided bacilli are sensitive) the speed of conversion is even greater. In the British Medical Research Council, studies on various chemotherapy regimens smear positive cases with usually advanced disease are enrolled. When such patients are given Isoniazid and Rifampin, 73 percent of them convert by the end of the second month and 94 percent by the end of the third month(52).

With Rifampin containing regimens, one often observes that smears are positive for a little longer than cultures. Such bacilli are considered nonviable.

The fact that sputum conversion almost invariably occurs in the first few months of treatment can be utilized in developing countries. In such countries standardized, inexpensive drug regimens have to be used in treatment and there are frequently no facilities and no resources for conducting sensitivity studies. At the same time, the prevalence of bacterial resistance is relatively high. If the sputum examination five or six months after commencement of therapy still shows tubercle bacilli this may be taken as evidence that this particular patient has a resistant infection and therefore there is no point in continuing with the current chemotherapy; the treatment should be changed to an alternative regimen if such is available.

BACTERIAL RESISTANCE

Resistance of tubercle bacilli to antimicrobial drugs is of great importance. The resistance is called "primary" when a patient is infected with bacilli already resistant to one or more antimicrobial agents or "secondary" when resistance is the result of previous faulty treatment, whether the fault was due to poor regimen prescribed or due to a poorly compliant patient taking drugs in an erroneous manner, e.g., one drug at a time.

Methods of establishing sensitivity of tubercle bacilli to anti-tuberculous drugs vary. Firstly, it is possible, when the specimens contain numerous bacilli to perform "direct" sensitivity tests by simply inoculating the specimens on various drug containing and drug free media. The indirect sensitivity tests, in which inoculates consist of cultures are much more commonly used. There are three methods of indirect sensitivity tests: the absolute concentration method, the resistance ratio method used in Britain and the proportion method where results show percentages of resistant organisms in the total bacterial population.

There is little doubt that primary resistance is more common in developing countries than in the developed countries. There are at least three good reasons for it. The first one is epidemiological. In the countries with low rates of tuberculosis the current risk of tuberculous infection is very small. Therefore, most of the cases of active tuberculosis tend to arise from infections acquired many years ago, frequently from those occuring before the introduction of antimicrobial treatment. Conversely, in countries with large tuberculosis problem a higher proportion of the total cases arise as a result of relatively recent primary infection, and therefore have a greater chance of being infected with resistant bacilli. Secondly, in such countries with a large tuberculosis problem and low financial resources, rather inadequate treatment was frequently given, particularly in the early years of chemotherapy. Monotherapy, with Isoniazid alone, was sometimes used and while admittedly it saved a lot of lives and affected many permanent cures, it resulted in an increase of acquired resistance followed by the increase in primary resistance. Inappropriate tuberculous drug regimens are also sometimes prescribed by private practitioners and sometimes Isoniazid is apparently added to cough mixtures and similar medications. Thirdly, some patients who received chemotherapy, previously, deny it, fearing that this may disqualify them from further treatment. This happens more commonly in developing countries and therefore figures for primary resistance may be somewhat exaggerated. Even when all these facts are taken into consideration it is quite obvious that certain countries, particularly western countries with little immigration, have very low primary resistance rates. For instance, Switzerland reports that only 1.3 percent of patients show primary resistance to Isoniazid, U.S.A. reports 4.4 percent of such patients, while Morocco reports 16.8 percent: all these studies were done in the 1970's. Before that, it was reported from Taiwan that in the 1968 prevalence survey, 26.9 percent of bacteriologically proven patients showed resistance to Isoniazid.

A survey of secondary resistance done periodically is very worthwhile. When such secondary resistance rises, obviously something is wrong with the treatment program; it should show a progressive fall as our knowledge of chemotherapy improves. With modern treatment regimens even non-compliant patients should not become resistant.

INFECTIVITY OF TUBERCULOSIS

Tuberculosis in the lay and sometimes even in the professional mind is often considered to be very infectious. For instance, the author was consulted recently on treatment of a case of tuberculous salpingitis in one of the local hospitals; the patient in question had no other manifestation of tuberculous disease yet strict isolation has been enforced; she obviously could not possibly infect anyone around her. Patients with any extrapulmonary form of disease are not infectious.

How infectious is a case of pulmonary tuberculosis? Table 6 is taken from a large study on contacts which the author and his colleagues conducted in two provinces of Canada, Saskatchewan and British Columbia. This table clearly shows that it is smear positive

TABLE 6

TUBERCULIN STATUS OF 1273 WHITE CHILDREN (0–9) LIVING WITH PATIENTS WITH ACTIVE PULMONARY TUBERCULOSIS— BRITISH COLUMBIA & SASKATCHEWAN 1966–1971

Bacteriological Status of Source		Positive Tuberculin Percent
Smear Positive	(640)	32.7
Culture Positive	(350)	9.1
Negative	(283)	6.3

cases of pulmonary tuberculosis who are the real sources of infection. With almost one third of young contacts of such smear positive cases becoming infected. Thus, even such cases are not very infectious. The percentage of positive reactors among contacts of the sources whose sputum was positive on culture only, with smears being negative and those clinical cases of active tuberculosis whose sputum was negative, both on smear and culture showed tuberculin positive rates well below 10 percent.

It can be concluded from these observations that tuberculosis is not a very infectious disease and that for practical purposes infectivity is confined to those advanced pulmonary cases whose sputum is positive on microscopic examination. Even in those cases, infectivity is not very high.

There are certain exceptions to this rule relating to patients whose sputum is literally teeming with bacilli and who cough and do not take precautions to cover the mouth when coughing. A case was described by Dr. Barnett of the Province of Saskatchewan of an Indian grandmother who decided to visit at Christmas time numerous members of her family, scattered throughout the province. Dr. Barnett followed her some three months later with the investigating team; the lady was apparently responsible for at least 13 cases of tuberculosis.

Thus, there is an occasional "Typhoid Mary" in tuberculosis. On the other hand, a distinguished physician, now dead for many years, had chronic bacillary tuberculosis in the pre-antimicrobial era with recurrent though not continuous positive sputum smears for a period of over 20 years. Yet, his two daughters who were in close contact with him throughout this period remained uninfected; all it took were reasonable but by no means excessive precautions on his part.

Infectivity of tuberculosis diminishes rapidly after the diagnosis is made, and antimicrobial treatment started. This is accounted for by rapidly diminishing bacterial population in the sputum and also by patient education about means of preventing infectivity.

There was another interesting observation made through analysis of the results of our study on contacts. This is shown in Table 7, and relates to morbidity, which in this table is calculated not only among all contacts but also among those who were infected (positive tuberculin reactors). It is obvious that morbidity among infected contacts of smear positive cases is much higher than that among similar contacts of smear negative cases. Thus, for some reason, smear positive cases not only infect those around them more frequently, but infect them more dangerously; this is possibly related to the dose of bacilli received at primary infection.

TABLE 7

ACTIVE TUBERCULOSIS AMONG 2130 WHITE CHILDREN 0-14 YEARS LIVING WITH PATIENTS WITH ACTIVE PULMONARY TUBERCULOSIS B.C. and SASK., 1966-71

Bacteriological Status of Source	Percent with Active Disease	
	All of Contacts	Those Infected (Tbn Pos)
Smear Positive	11.3	37.7
Culture Positive	1.7	18.2
Negative	0.6	9.7

CHAPTER XV

NATURAL HISTORY OF TUBERCULOSIS IN THE COMMUNITY: EPIDEMIOLOGY OF TUBERCULOSIS

Tuberculosis is still a major health problem in the world. A very conservative estimate based on the known incidence rates indicates that there are at least 8 million bacteriologically confirmed cases of tuberculosis diagnosed in the world every year. The number of cases, which are never diagnosed is obviously unknown but is possibly only a little less than that of diagnosed cases.

Tuberculosis is very unevenly distributed. This is illustrated in Figure 7 for a few selected countries. It is quite clear that the overall rates are low in Canada and in the U.S.

In 1977, over 30,000 cases were diagnosed and notified in the United States, giving a rate of 13.9 per 100,000. The corresponding number of active cases notified in Canada was just over 3000, a rate of 13.7/100,000.

The rates in other countries are often higher. In Taiwan, for instance, the rate is 39.4/100,000, in Columbia 89.0/100,000 and in the Philippines 328/100,000. It is clear that we are dealing here with a spectrum of rates rather than with a clear cut division between low and high prevalence countries.

Even in Canada and the United States, the distribution of the tuberculosis problem is quite uneven between different groups of population. This is illustrated in Figure 8.

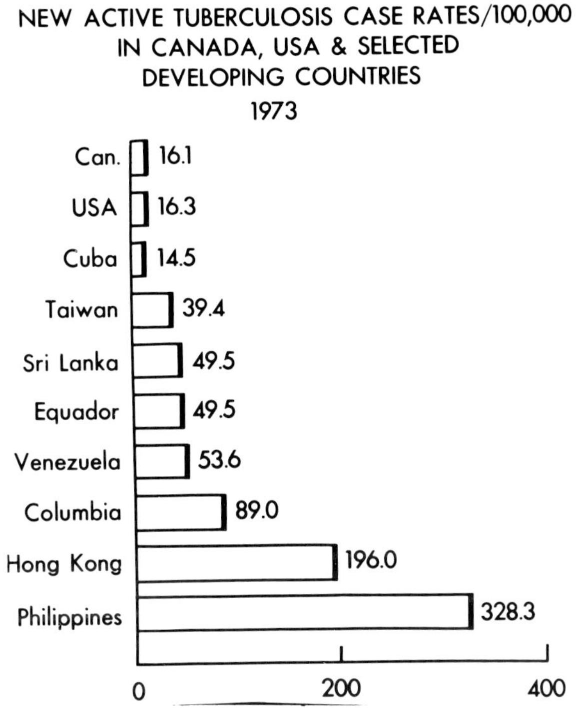

Figure 7. New active tuberculosis case rates per 100,000 in Canada, U.S.A. and selected developing countries 1973.

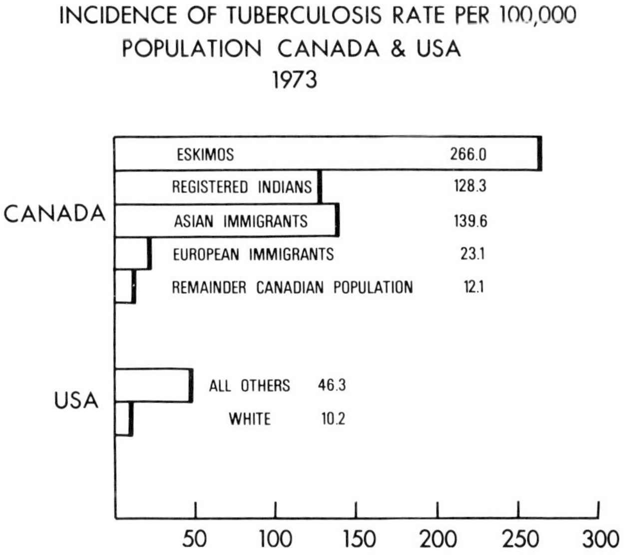

Figure 8. Incidence of tuberculosis, rates per 100,000 Canada and U.S.A. 1973.

TUBERCULOSIS MORTALITY

The introduction of antimicrobial drugs to the treatment of tuberculosis in the 1950's has very dramatically reduced the mortality from this disease. Figure 9 illustrates this for Canada and the United States. While prior to the introduction of antimicrobial drugs, there has been a steady decline for many decades, the rate dropped dramatically in the early 1950's and a steep decline continued through the 1960's and the 1970's, recently showing a slight tendency towards slowing down. In recent years, the mortality rate in both countries has been about one-tenth of the incidence rate. In the pre-antimicrobial days, the mortality rate was roughly half the morbidity rate; in old days, if one developed pulmonary tuberculosis—the main form of the disease—the chances of death over the next few years were about 50:50.

With the dramatic decline of the mortality rate in the United States and Canada to a level of just over 1 per 100,000 in the late 1970's, it was realized that a substantial proportion (often more than half) of the deaths from tuberculosis are due to failure of diagnosis during life. As Table 8 indicates, this failure of diagnosis is particularly common in the case of two forms of disease; miliary tuberculosis and tuberculous meningitis. In Canada, almost a quarter of the cases of miliary tuberculosis were first diagnosed after death; the same was

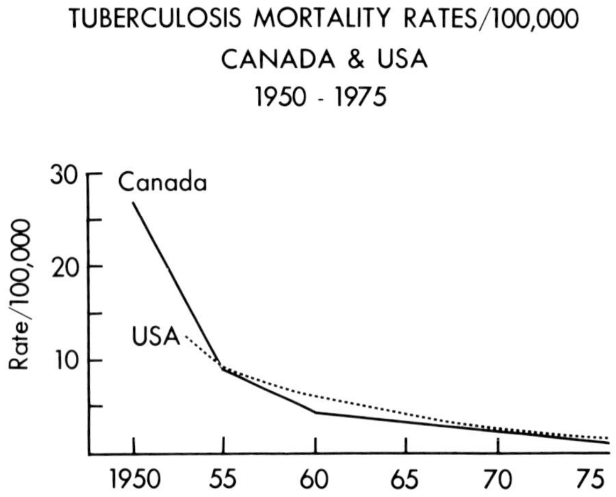

Figure 9. Tuberculosis mortality rates per 100,000 Canada and U.S.A. 1950–1975.

TABLE 8

TUBERCULOSIS FIRST REPORTED AT DEATH
PERCENT OF CASES

	Canada 1970–1974	United States 1969–1973
Miliary	22.6	29.7
Meningitis	14.5	22.7

true for close to 15 percent of cases of meningitis. In the United States during the corresponding period, the situation was even a little worse. In Canada at least, the proportion of deaths from this highly curable disease diagnosed for the first time after death is increasing. Most of these cases diagnosed after death actually came to light at postmortem examination. In a few, diagnosis is suspected before death but positive bacteriological reports do not come until after the patient's demise. The number of such cases diagnosed after death is obviously related to the autopsy rate in the area. In British Columbia, for instance, about one-third of all deaths come to autopsy—a relatively high rate. It appears not unreasonable to expect that tuberculosis is present and is the cause of death in some of the remaining two-thirds of deaths in whom autopsy is not carried out. Obviously, the problem of diagnosis of cases dying from unrecognised tuberculosis points to the lack of awareness of this diagnostic possibility in some severely ill patients with complex clinical problems. The remedy for this tragic situation lies in better medical education.

MORBIDITY—AGE AND SEX

Figure 10 shows age and sex specific annual incidence rates in Canada and the U.S. It is quite clear that up to the age of about 30 years tuberculosis is relatively uncommon, the rates rising from about 5 per 100,000 to 18 per 100,000; there are also no differences between the two sexes. Later on in life, rates for men continue to rise, reaching close to 70 per 100,000 in older men over the age of 65. The rates in the females on the whole stay around 20 per 100,000 throughout their life with possibly a slight rise in elderly women.

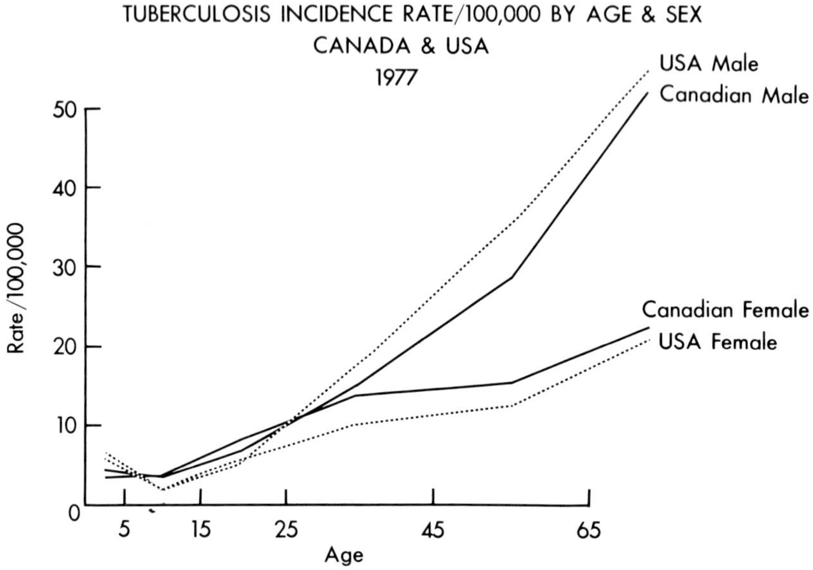

Figure 10. Age-sex specific annual tuberculosis incidence rates per 100,000 Canada and U.S.A. 1977.

The shape of the curves depicting tuberculosis rates was not always like that. A hundred years ago the shape of the curves was quite different; the rates were highest in early adult life, particularly among women, similar to that seen among Canadian Eskimos in the Eastern Arctic in the 1960's (Figure 11). The evolution from the disease predominantly affecting young women to that predominant in old men is well documented in the so-called cohort analysis of tuberculosis mortality(53). It is beyond the scope of this book to go into details of this analysis, suffice to say that in all the communities in which tuberculosis is declining, and it is declining almost everywhere in the world, the rate of this decline is much faster in the younger than in the older age groups. The shape of the curves depicting tuberculosis rates as seen in Canada or the United States, (Figure 10), is by itself a byproduct or a sign of decline. Post-primary pulmonary tuberculosis is by its very nature primarily a disease of young adults particularly the young women; it is almost certainly the steady decline in the intensity of tuberculous infection which accounts for the continuous change in the age and sex specific rates.

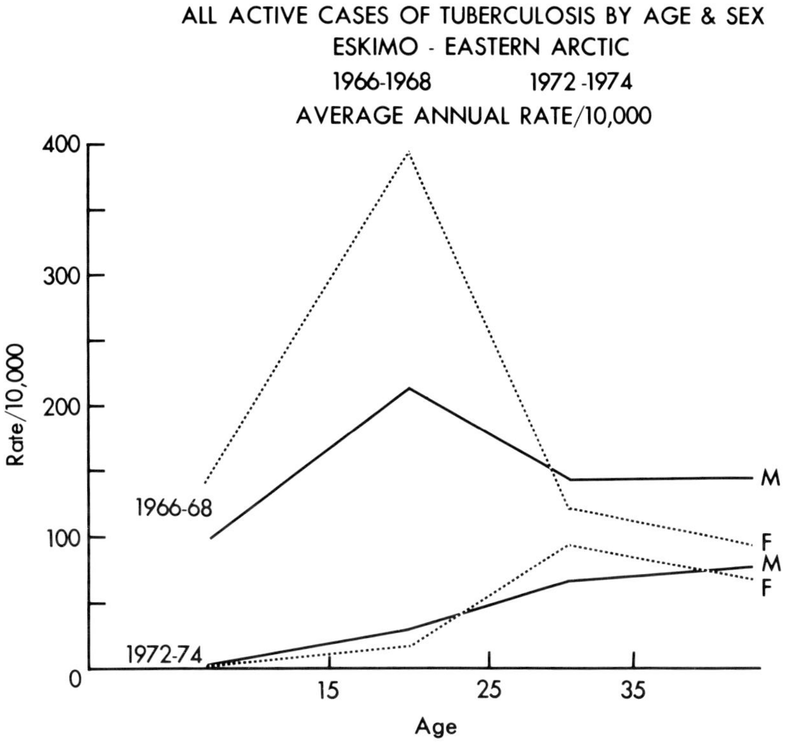

Figure 11. All active cases of tuberculosis by age and sex. Average annual rates per 10,000. Eskimos Eastern Arctic 1966–1968 and 1972–1974.

Decline of Tuberculosis: As already stated, tuberculosis is declining slowly but steadily (Fig. 12) throughout most of the world today. The calculated rate of decline in the late 1960's and 1970's in Canada is about 5 percent per annum. In the Canadian Eskimos, where the rates were extremely high, an intensive tuberculosis control program was launched in the 1960's. This resulted in an unprecedented rate of decline of over 16 percent annually. It is difficult to be sure as to how much of the decline of tuberculosis in any given country is due to control program and how much is due to the natural behavior of this disease. Probably a reasonable estimate of natural decline would be around 2 percent per annum for most countries; the balance is accounted for by tuberculosis program. If the present rate of decline of

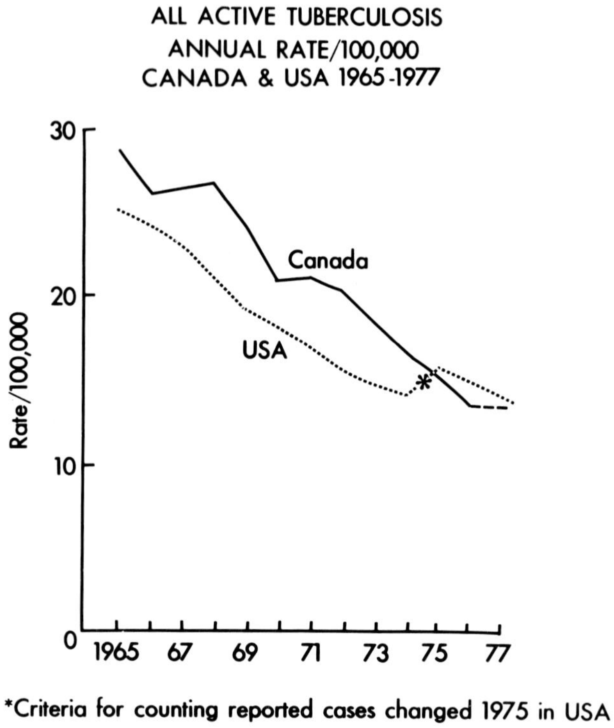

Figure 12. All active tuberculosis annual rates per 100,000 Canada and United States 1965–1977.

5 percent continues in Canada, our number of cases, which is now just over 3,000 will decline to 2,000 by 1990 and to 1,200 by the year 2000. The number of cases in the United States in those years is likely to be about ten times greater.

TUBERCULOSIS IN IMMIGRANTS

One of the interesting features of a study of tuberculosis in immigrants relates to the fact that the rates of tuberculosis among different groups are closer to those seen in their country of origin than to those of the country in which they have settled. Table 9 illustrates this point. The rates of tuberculosis among immigrants from various countries, are, while similar, generally somewhat lower than those seen in their country of origin. This is accounted for, at least in part,

TABLE 9

TUBERCULOSIS MORBIDITY AMONG RESIDENTS IN CANADA BORN IN OTHER COUNTRIES 1970–1972

Country of Birth	Incidence Rate (Per 100,000 Population)	
	In Country of Birth	In Canada
Philippines	300	219.5
Finland	98.8	77.6
Scandinavia (Excl. Fin)	17.9	26.0
Greece	106.9	42.3
Austria	66.5	32.1
United Kingdom	25.3	15.5
Canada	—	15.5

by the quite careful screening of the immigrant population for tuberculosis. Perhaps the most dramatic illustration of the fact that immigrants bring, as it were, the tuberculosis problem from the "old" country is the difference between the rates among the Finns in Canada and those among other Scandinavians. Finland has three times the rate of tuberculosis than that in the other Scandinavian countries and the same ratio is seen in Finns and other Scandinavians living in Canada. This is in spite of the fact that the average period of stay in Canada for both the Finnish and other Scandinavian cases is over 40 years(54).

TUBERCULOSIS INFECTION RATES

Tuberculin surveys of the general population particularly of younger segments of populations have become quite popular since the 1950's. The stimulus for these surveys arose from the quite surprising finding that in many developed countries the percentage of positive reactors was appreciably lower than expected at the time. The author conducted extensive tuberculin surveys in the province of Ontario, Canada(55), and was able to show that the rates in the population of that province were generally low (Figure 13). Low rates in children obviously indicate that there has not been much tuberculous infection around for some years; rising rates in middle age reflect

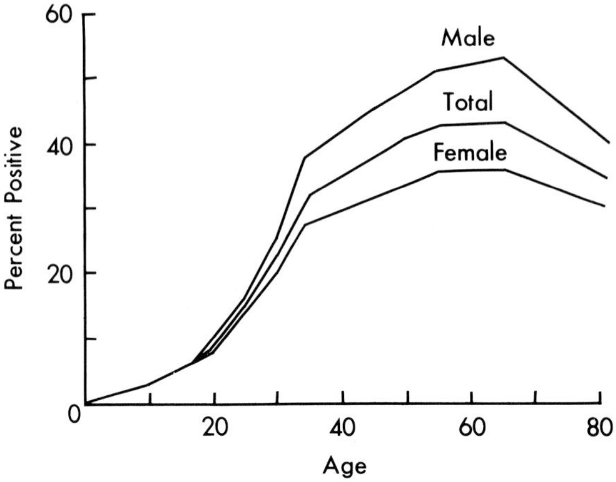

Figure 13. Tuberculin testing, Ontario—male and female.

mainly remote infection; there was a much higher risk of infection some decades earlier. The fall in the rates in the elderly seen in practically every tuberculin survey of the population must be artificial, probably indicating an impaired ability of the elderly to react to the low dose of tuberculin.

Figure 14 shows the differences in results of tuberculin tests between Ontario and Taiwan, obviously the differences are profound; by the age of 20 less than 20 percent of individuals in Ontario and close to 80 percent of individuals in Taiwan showed a positive reaction to tuberculin. These differences reflect a much greater tuberculosis problem in Taiwan than in Ontario.

It is also interesting to observe the differences between various groups of population. Figure 15 from the Ontario study shows that North American Indians have high rates as compared to Canadian born individuals with immigrants falling in between. Differences between the Indian and Canadian born segments of the population reflect the different tuberculosis problems. As measured by morbidity and mortality rates Canadian Indians have always had some ten times more tuberculosis than Canadian-born whites. The same was not true however when one compared the differences between foreign-born and Canadian-born groups. After age adjustment, the foreign-born (at the time of this study the vast majority of them were born in Europe) had a much smaller tuberculosis problem than the differences between the two tuberculin curves would lead one to expect.

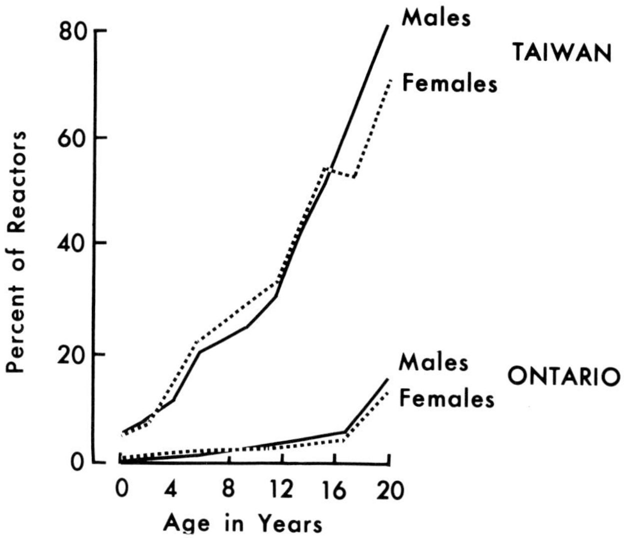

Figure 14. Tuberculin sensitivity Ontario and Taiwan.

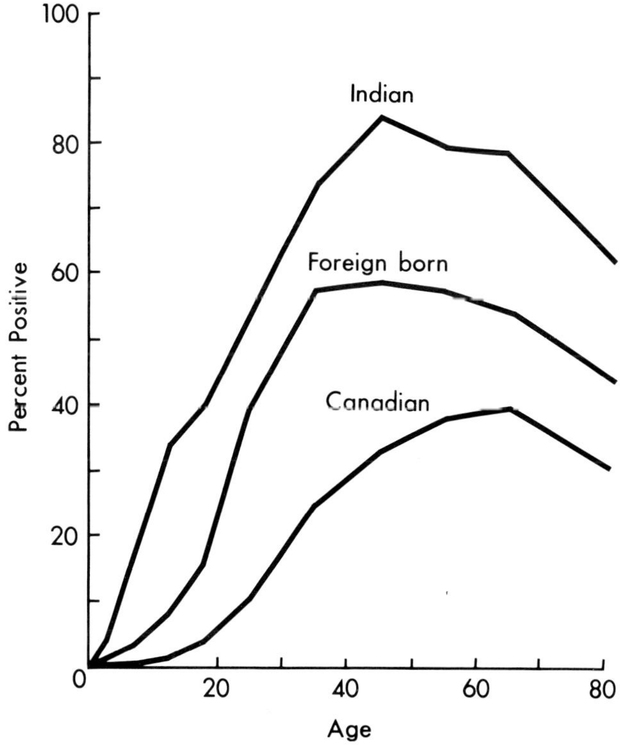

Figure 15. Tuberculin testing, Ontario—Registered Indian, Foreign-born, Other Canadian-born.

The uncertainties of the tuberculin reaction have been discussed extensively earlier in this book. It is not difficult to explain why tuberculin positive rates in the population do not reflect accurately the tuberculosis morbidity and mortality rates. Tuberculin positive individuals seen in such surveys consist of differing proportions of:
1) Those recently infected—high-risk situation.
2) Those remotely infected with tubercle bacilli—low-risk situation.
3) Those infected with atypical mycobacteria—no or even negative (because of BCG like effect) risk situation. In addition, individuals with negative reaction as seen in such surveys include "revertors" to the particular dose of tuberculin; this group presumably carries a small risk of disease.

It can be concluded that while tuberculin surveys are useful from the epidemiological point of view, showing gross differences between the tuberculosis problem in various populations, they are not a very precise epidemiological index.

CHAPTER XVI

ATYPICAL (NON-TUBERCULOUS) MYCOBACTERIA

It is logical to consider atypical mycobacteria in a book on tuberculosis as they have several important interactions with the tuberculosis problem.

First, they sometimes render interpretation of the tuberculin reaction difficult. This was discussed at length in the chapter on tuberculin testing, suffice to recall here that many small and medium sized reactions to the 5 TU PPD tuberculin are often caused by infections with atypical mycobacteria. Individuals infected with these organisms sometimes react to tuberculin with the same size of reaction as individuals infected with tubercle bacilli. The dividing line between what should be considered true positive reaction (specific to infection with tubercle bacilli) and what is a non-specific reaction (due to infections with atypical mycobacteria) is impossible to draw accurately. In the Vancouver area, for instance, in young people where infections with atypical mycobacteria are relatively common, while those with tubercle bacilli are quite uncommon, 25 percent of tuberculin reactions between 10 and 14 mm and 13 percent of those between 15 and 19 mm were found to be non-specific(56). These were studies done by dual testing with 5 TU PPD-S and with an equivalent dose of Gause antigen PPD-G. Obviously, if one can imagine a community in which there is no longer any tuberculous infection then all tuberculin reactions independent of size would be due to atypical infections. Conversely, in communities in which tuberculous infection is still very common the majority of reactions, whether over or under an arbitrary diameter of 10 mm are likely to be due to tuberculous infection.

We estimated that in our area, if everybody was infected with atypical mycobacteria and nobody with tubercle bacilli then based on the 10 mm criterion of reaction to 5 TU of PPD-S, 10 percent of individuals would be considered positive tuberculin reactors.

Secondly, atypical mycobacterial infections provide a degree of acquired resistance to infections with tubercle bacilli. This has been shown by a number of experimental studies(57) and in an epidemiological investigation of U.S. Navy recruits(74). This effect of atypical mycobacterial infection is similar but usually less pronounced than that produced by BCG vaccination.

DISEASES DUE TO ATYPICAL MYCOBACTERIA

Atypical mycobacteria are truly reluctant pathogens and we have estimated that their pathogenicity is some 40 times lower than that of tubercle bacilli(58). It therefore appears extremely unlikely as suggested by some, that disease caused by these organisms will ever achieve an importance comparable to that of tuberculosis.

Although atypical mycobacteriosis may probably occur in any organ affected by tuberculosis, disease is seen most commonly at three sites: the lungs, cervical lymph nodes and more rarely skin. It should be realized that although for purposes of this discussion all "pathogenic" atypical mycobacteria are grouped together, each of them has different disease producing potential and differs in epidemiological and clinical aspects. They also differ greatly in sensitivity to antimicrobial agents.

1) Pulmonary Atypical Mycobacteriosis: This is the most common form of the disease and clinically and radiologically it closely resembles or perhaps is identical with post-primary pulmonary tuberculosis. In our series of cases, due to *Mycobacterium intracellulare—Avium complex*—the disease is twice as common in men than in women. In some series in which the disease is predominantly due to *Mycobacterium kansasii,* male to female ratio may be as high as 9 to 1. The disease attacks predominantly elderly people and predisposing conditions are the same as those discussed in the case of post-primary pulmonary tuberculosis.

In the diagnosis of this disease, the *repeated* isolation of the same organism from the sputum of a patient with radiological picture compatible with tuberculosis is essential. Single scanty isolation of atypical mycobacteria in the sputum are quite common and are usually of no significance whatsoever. Skin testing with PPD-S and atypical antigens is rarely helpful diagnostically in the pulmonary form of disease. Occasionally, completely negative reactions are obtained; in those who are positive, the distinction in sizes of reactions elicited by different antigens is often not as clear cut as that in children.

The course of the disease is often protracted, even perhaps more so than was seen in tuberculosis in the pre-antimicrobial era. Remissions are usually quite prolonged but are commonly followed by spread of the disease.

In cases due to *M. intracellulare*—avium complex—antimicrobial treatment in the author's judgment is ineffective although some authorities report some success with multiple drug regimens.(59,60) We have tried to use transfer factor in some of our patients but could not really detect any improvement. Patients with other atypical bacilli are more fortunate, such as those with diseases due to *Mycobacterium kansasii,* as their bacilli are sensitive to at least some of the antituberculous drugs. Well localized disease maybe resected but various post-surgical complications are common.

2) Cervical Adenitis: This has already been discussed. In British Columbia, at least, all our cases are young white children coming from well-to-do homes. Most of them live in a low lying area of the city with a lot of marshland and extensive shoreline. Most of the cases here are due to the organism belonging to *M. intracellulare—avium* type. Usually, a single gland lying just behind the angle of the jaw is involved. The outlook for these cases is excellent and no real treatment is available or necessary. Surgery is usually performed for diagnosis which is, of course, only definitely established if the offending mycobacterium is isolated; unfortunately the whole specimen is often placed in preservative. Skin testing with PPD tuberculin (5TU equivalent) and corresponding atypical antigens are quite helpful in this group, all showing much larger reactions to Gause and Battey antigen than to PPD-S.

3) Swimming pool granuloma due to *M. balnei* is seen occasionally; on the parts liable to abrasions while swimming, e.g., knees. Similar condition is sometimes seen in aquarium owners and rarely in fishermen. It is of interest that the program of building swimming pools in schools in Norway has affected the results of tuberculin surveys of students.

CHAPTER XVII

PREVENTIVE PROGRAMS

STRATEGY OF TUBERCULOSIS CONTROL

In its broad concept this strategy is applicable to all countries, poor or rich, developing or developed. It is based on tuberculosis programs; we can divide these programs into curative and preventive (Table 10). The curative program consists of case finding and treatment. These two programs should really be considered as one for obviously case finding does not make sense unless we cure the cases we find. This was sometimes forgotten and in some countries in the past the case finding outstripped the capacity of treatment programs. The two preventive programs are quite distinct: BCG vaccination and chemoprophylaxis. The first of these is applicable to uninfected tuberculin negative individuals with a high risk of infection. Chemoprophylaxis is used primarily for individuals already infected; its purpose is to diminish the chances of developing the disease.

TABLE 10

STRATEGY OF TUBERCULOSIS PROGRAMS

	"Curative"	**Preventive**
Aims	Reduction of deaths and suffering	Reduction of future morbidity and infection
	Reduction of current TB infection	
Programs	Case finding	BCG
	Treatment	Chemoprophylaxis

The effect of the "curative" program is reduction of deaths and suffering. From the epidemiological point of view, it reduces current tuberculous infection. The impact of the case finding–treatment program is immediate; it therefore has the most powerful influence on the tuberculosis problem.

Both the preventive programs reduce morbidity and risk of infection in the future, sometimes in the quite distant future. Their contribution to the reduction of tuberculosis problem in the community is therefore less important because it is more remote.

CASE FINDING

There are three diagnostic tools—tuberculin test, chest x-ray and bacteriological examination by smear and culture. They have already been discussed at length. As far as the tuberculin test is concerned, suffice to say that while not denying the usefulness of this simple test in many clinical situations, we have likely been guilty in North America of over-emphasizing its value in tuberculosis control. Some 20 years ago, the author was a very great enthusiast in applying this test widely in tuberculosis programs. As years went by, the limitation of the tuberculin test became increasingly obvious and it became apparent that it is a poor screening test. This is due to the fact that many positive reactions are due to infections with atypical mycobacteria or to BCG vaccination. Furthermore, in order to eliminate false positive reactions, we use such a small dose of tuberculin that we get many "false negative" reactions; between 5–14 percent of our cases of bacillary tuberculosis do not give a positive reaction to 5 T.U. It is an inexpensive test. Tuberculin test is of course of considerable value in special clinical situations, for instance in examination of young contacts of a case of tuberculosis.

Chest x-ray was considered, until recently, to be *the* important tool for diagnosis of tuberculosis. Its value has considerably decreased particularly in the communities where tuberculosis rates are low. Other diseases such as lung cancer or fungus infection are in some groups just as common as, if not commoner than tuberculosis, as a cause of shadowing which looks like tuberculosis. Under program situations chest x-ray is good as a screening tool for bacteriological examination. In many towns and cities in developing countries good mass x-ray equipment is available; it is often cheapest there to employ the chest x-ray as the first test and to examine bacteriologically only the x-ray suspects.

Bacteriological examination of sputum is obviously a most definitive test for pulmonary tuberculosis. As in many countries, the rate of bacteriological confirmation of pulmonary tuberculosis is of the order of 80 percent, there is no reason, as already discussed, why bacteriology should not be used as a primary diagnostic tool. Indeed, in many developing countries, microscopic examination of the sputum of patients reporting to primary health units with symptoms constitutes the main case finding program. The advantages of smear examination are that smears are easy to examine and cheap to prepare. Furthermore, really important sources of infection are diagnosed. Its disadvantage is that advanced cases are discovered by this method and such cases are more difficult to cure. There are also occasional false positive results; it is always wise in mass case-finding programs to have the diagnosis established by two positive findings, be it two positive smears or a positive smear and a positive culture or a positive smear and a compatible chest x-ray.

Culture examination is more expensive than microscopy. Its other disadvantage is the delay of six weeks. Its great advantage is that the disease is usually diagnosed in a less advanced stage; it is easier to cure and does not lead to extensive residual damage.

TREATMENT PROGRAM

Treatment of tuberculosis has been discussed in detail elsewhere; here certain factors relating to mass chemotherapy programs operating particularly in the developing countries will be emphasized. Treatment is the most difficult, costly and often the weakest of the tuberculosis programs. This is due to two factors, firstly there are uncooperative patients; to use the World Health Organization term "defaulters." Secondly inappropriate regimens are still often prescribed in some countries. It is now perfectly possible to make tuberculosis treatment quite effective provided three conditions are met.

1) Potent drug regimens capable of curing the vast majority of patients are utilized.

Such a drug regimen must take into account the existing resistance pattern of tubercle bacilli in the particular country. This, in practice, means utilization of Rifampin as one of the drugs used in routine treatment. In spite of its expense, it will in a long run prove the cheapest way of combating the problem of tuberculosis. Apart from high cure rate, the aim of such drug regimen must be to decrease and not to increase the prevalence of resistant organisms in the population.

2) The regimen should be of short duration to assure better acceptability and fewer defaulters.

3) Treatment must be completely supervised; this usually requires the utilization of intermittent regimens.

It is the author's firm belief that the countries adopting the above principles in their treatment programs will truly control their tuberculosis and witness an accelerated decline of this disease.

BCG VACCINATION

Sixty years ago, Calmette and Guerin produced BCG Vaccine through attenuation of bovine bacilli by prolonged cultivation on glycerol-potato medium. It was in 1921 that the first French child was vaccinated. Since that time, many millions of people all around the world have received this vaccine.

BCG received a major setback in the form of the Lübeck tragedy in 1930 when the 251 newborn infants received by mistake virulent human bacilli; 72 of them died of tuberculosis. However, by the time of the Second World War, BCG had re-established its reputation as a valuable and almost completely harmless immunizing agent. Since the war it had been accepted and widely used in almost every country with the exception of North America. In England, there were originally a lot of misgivings about injecting into human beings a living agent. However, after the war and particularly after the first results of the British Medical Research Council trial, BCG vaccination was accepted as an official program for "school leavers."

Objections to BCG in the United States stem from two factors. The first is an erroneous hypothesis on the pathogenesis of post-primary pulmonary tuberculosis; according to this hypothesis, post-primary tuberculosis arises as a result of re-infection of tissues rendered "allergic" by previous primary infection(61). Were it true we would obviously find that BCG vaccinated subjects develop tuberculosis more frequently and in more severe forms. Although there is considerable variation in assessment of protective powers of BCG, nobody has shown that BCG produces such deleterious effects. The second objection stems from the fact that BCG vaccination renders the tuberculin reaction positive and therefore destroys the value of tuberculin testing in tuberculosis control programs and epidemiological studies. This objection is valid, but as discussed elsewhere the value of the tuberculin test and particularly of the programs relying on periodical repetition of tuberculin tests is already grossly undermined by the atypical mycobacterial infections.

EFFECTIVENESS OF BCG VACCINATION

There were several major BCG trials in the world and Sutherland gave a thoughtful review of seven of them(62). Since that time, results of a large trial in southern India have been published. They show no protective value of BCG in that particular population(63). Protection derived from BCG varied between 80 and 0 percent (Table 11). It is now generally agreed that these differences in the protective power of BCG are due to two factors. Firstly, there is differing prevalence of atypical mycobacterial infections in the areas where the trials were conducted and these infections act as natural vaccination. BCG in areas with high prevalence of such infections is therefore given to already partly immunized subjects. Secondly, the immunogenic properties of different vaccines vary a great deal.

As already stated, apart from the United States, Canada and a few European countries (e.g., the Netherlands) mass vaccination programs exist in practically every country and in most countries BCG vaccination is compulsory. The author reviewed the data(64) from 14 African and 24 Asian countries, with a total population of 1¼ billion. In one year alone (1968), over 31 million vaccinations were given in those countries.

TABLE 11

SUMMARY INFORMATION OF TEN CONTROLLED TRIALS OF BCG VACCINATION AGAINST TUBERCULOSIS

Trial	Reference	Duration of Observation (Years)	Percent Protection
North America Indians (62)	Stein & Aronson 1953	9–11	80
Chicago Infants (62)	Rosenthal et al 1961	12–23	75
Georgia School Children (62)	Comstock & Webster 1969	20	Nil
Puerto Rico Children (62)	Palmer et al 1958	6–8	31
Georgia & Alabama Population (62)	Comstock & Palmer 1966	14	14
Britain School Children (62)	Medical Research Council 1971	15	78
S. India Rural Population (62)	Frimodt-Moller et al 1964	3–7	60
Saskatchewan Nurses (72)	Ferguson 1955	1–14	80
Saskatchewan Sanitoria Employees (72)	Ferguson 1955	1–14	85
S. India Population (63)	Tuberculosis Prevention Trial Madras 1980	7½	Nil

TIME OF VACCINATION

In some countries, vaccination of newborns and infants is widely practised. In some (e.g., Britain), the age of first vaccination is postponed until early adolescence (school leavers). In most, vaccination is given throughout childhood, sometimes repeatedly. Deliberate re-vaccination in adolescence is often practised. The main value of vaccinating the newborns is protection from severe hematogenous forms of tuberculosis, particularly from meningitis. Vaccination in adolescence on the other hand protects against development of post-primary pulmonary tuberculosis; it is therefore of greater epidemiological importance as it may reduce the number of new sources of infection arising in the community.

METHOD OF VACCINATION

The intradermal method of vaccination is adopted in most countries. The technique is identical with that employed in the Mantoux test; the site of injection is usually the skin over the deltoid muscle. In some countries, various per-cutaneous methods are used (including scratch and modified Heaf gun); in Brazil, oral vaccination has been extensively practised. In most vaccination programs, freeze-dried BCG is used as it is much longer lasting than liquid preparations.

It is unfortunate that there are many different BCG's produced in the world; it sometimes seems that for a country to develop its own BCG laboratory is a status symbol.

Pre-vaccination tuberculin test consisting usually of 5 TU (occasionally 250 TU is also used) is done in all developed countries and only negative reactors are vaccinated. In some developing countries, for organizational reasons, direct vaccination, without a previous tuberculin test is practised; no untoward effects of such an approach are reported. Post-vaccination tests are done routinely in some areas. They are generally unnecessary and inspection of vaccination site suffices. However, post-vaccination tuberculin tests should always be done in a sample of vaccinated with a new batch of the vaccine. BCG scar occurs in most individuals vaccinated by intradermal method; it is a smaller and deeper scar than that arising from smallpox vaccination.

COMPLICATIONS OF BCG VACCINATION

A small local ulcer is almost invariable and should not be considered as a complication; it usually heals after a period of some weeks. Axillary lympadenitis is probably the most common complication. It occurs more frequently when a stronger vaccine or a larger dose is used; it is also more frequent in infants than in older children. Bone lesions have been described in Scandinavia and there is currently an international investigation trying to delineate their frequency. Keloid formation appears to be particularly common in Oriental children following re-vaccination. Deaths due to BCG are few (less than one in a million vaccinated)—they are probably all due to vaccination of immunologically incompetent individuals. Very large doses of BCG are now used in treatment of malignancies and even here serious complications are few.

EFFICACY

The efficacy of vaccination is very difficult to measure under ordinary program conditions. However, one way of getting some idea of the value of the BCG program in developing countries is to look for the presence of BCG scar in children under the age of 5 who suffer from tuberculous meningitis. The frequency of such scars can then be compared with a group of controls matched for age. The author learned this approach in Taiwan where considerable protection from BCG was demonstrated (only 3.7 percent of cases of meningitis showed BCG scars against 34 percent expected). Similar investigation in one of the South American republics apparently has shown no protective value from the BCG used there.

THE PLACE OF BCG VACCINATION IN TUBERCULOSIS CONTROL PROGRAM

In developing countries, particularly in those countries with no, or with only moderate, prevalence of atypical mycobacterial infections, BCG vaccination on a mass scale should be continued. In developed countries with a very low risk of tuberculous infection, mass vaccination should be abandoned. However, in many of such countries this will require a change of legislation as BCG is compulsory by law; such a change is often very slow. In all the developed countries, BCG should, however, be offered to groups with a high risk of tuberculous infection. Such groups in North America include:

1) Eskimos and Indians. All of the Eskimos and North American Indians in Canada receive vaccination in childhood.

2) Persons likely to come in contact with tuberculous patients such as nurses, medical students, physicians and other hospital staff. A

BCG program in these groups is more effective and less troublesome than the program relying on repeated tuberculin testing adopted by many hospitals in the United States. As already discussed, periodical surveillance with tuberculin test of the health personnel (e.g. hospital staff) is not only difficult to organize but often leads to unreliable and erroneous results. The pitfalls of tuberculin testing become particularly troublesome and numerous in programs relying on repetition of the tests.

3) Individuals leaving for a high-incidence area, particularly if they are likely to come into close contact with the population—e.g., Peace Corps Volunteers.

4) Tuberculin negative contacts of cases of tuberculosis; in many of these vaccination is probably unnecessary as sources of infections are usually completely cured nowadays. However, relapses are still not uncommon and tuberculosis often arises in the environment in which there is more than one potential or actual source of infection. Vaccination should be mandatory if the source case harbours resistant bacilli.

CHEMOPROPHYLAXIS

The main credit for introducing this valuable preventive program in tuberculosis control goes to the United States Public Health Service. Well designed and efficiently carried out chemoprophylaxis trials were conducted in a number of "high-risk" groups such as contacts, Eskimos in Alaska, patients in psychiatric institutions, inactive cases of tuberculosis, etc. The results of each of these studies were carefully reported. They were elegantly summarized by Ferebee in 1970(65). Later on, the International Union against Tuberculosis at the instigation of the U.S. Public Health Service conducted a large scale trial in Eastern European countries on the value of chemoprophylaxis in fibrotic lesions (extensive scarring in the lungs suggestive of healed lesions of postprimary pulmonary tuberculosis)(66). In comparison to these great efforts of the U.S. Public Health Service and I.U.A.T., the contribution of other investigators was more modest. The author and his colleagues conducted two studies on chemoprophylaxis, one on patients with inactive tuberculosis who had not received adequate chemotherapy in the past and another on Canadian Eskimos (67,69,75).

The results of all these trials are summarized in Table 12. It will be seen that chemoprophylaxis is effective, the degree of effectiveness varying from 100 percent to 17 percent. It is effective in individuals who have a very high but short-lived risk of tuberculous disease such as recently infected contacts, and in those who have a somewhat lower but sustained risk (fibrotic lesions). Furthermore, the effects of

TABLE 12

SUMMARY INFORMATION ON SEVEN CONTROLLED TRIALS OF CHEMOPROPHYLAXIS AGAINST TUBERCULOSIS

Group	Drugs	Follow-up	Effectiveness
Household Contacts USPHS Trial	INH—12 mos.	10 years	60%
Patients in Mental Institutions (USPHS Trial)	INH—12 mos.	10 years	
Positive Reactors			
a) Normal x-ray			70%
b) Abnormal x-ray			49%
Inactive Lesions USPHS Trial	INH—12 mos.	5 years	
a) Never known active			63%
b) Previous active untreated			51%
c) Previous active treated			17%
Inactive Lesions			
Previous Active untreated Canada	INH 6-18 mos.	11 years	70%
	INH/PAS 6-18 mos.	11 years	90%
Alaska Villagers USPHS Trial	INH—12 mos.	6 years	59%
Greenland Villagers	INH twice a week for two periods of 3 months each	6 years	31%
Frobisher Bay Eskimos	INH/EMB 18 mos.	3 years	100%

chemoprophylaxis do not diminish with time. A twelve-month course of Isoniazid alone, is slightly superior to those of shorter duration, and an addition of another drug to Isoniazid probably renders chemoprophylaxis more effective and prevents a slight danger of Isoniazid resistance(69).

In the 1960's, it seemed we had a most powerful weapon against tuberculosis in our hands. We had a cheap, safe drug which could be taken by large number of people infected with tubercle bacilli, and had the potential for reducing the tuberculosis problem. We were aware of the epidemiological fact that perhaps as much as 80 percent of all active cases in North America arise as a result of remote infections and that if we could diminish the risk of tuberculous disease among those individuals infected a long time ago, by say 50 or 60 percent, we would achieve a great reduction of the total tuberculosis problem. Attempts were indeed made in certain areas to implement the policy of widespread chemoprophylaxis; in some states employees of large industrial plants were tuberculin tested and those with positive reaction were placed on Isoniazid for one year.

The enthusiasm for widespread chemoprophylaxis received the first blow by the realization that many, perhaps most individuals are by nature non-compliant and that considerable effort directed towards motivation and supervision would be necessary to ensure that they take the drug. Secondly, it seemed doubtful whether the relatively low risk such as that experienced for instance by the middle aged positive reactor (even if definitely infected with tubercle bacilli) warranted the effort involved. If the risk of developing tuberculosis by such an individual is for instance somewhere between one in a thousand to one in two thousand per annum, is it really worthwhile to take medication for one year in order to convert this risk to one in four thousand? In either case, such an individual is very unlikely to develop tuberculosis and if he develops it, it can be readily cured. Thirdly, the major blow to the idea of mass chemoprophylaxis came from the Baltimore tragedy where 13 people died from hepatitis, presumably induced by Isoniazid(70). As a result of all these, really widespread chemoprophylaxis used as a major public health preventive measure was no longer possible.

This is not to say that this powerful preventive measure should be abandoned altogether; however, its use should be confined to individuals with a really high risk of developing tuberculosis. As we have to weigh the benefits of chemoprophylaxis against sizeable disadvantages, the benefits have to be quite substantial.

What are the disadvantages of INH chemoprophylaxis? First is Isoniazid toxicity mainly but not entirely INH-induced hepatitis. In addition to this serious but fortunately rare complication there are occasional allergic reactions as well as the effects of this drug on the central and peripheral nervous systems. There have been suspicions that children taking Isoniazid do not do as well at school as those not taking the drug; there is also a possibility of neuropathy when malnutrition coexists. The second disadvantage of Isoniazid is the possibility of induction of Isoniazid resistance. This is probably quite real, particularly when Isoniazid is given to individuals with a sizeable bacterial population such as inactive cases. In the Canadian study two of 12 bacteriologically confirmed relapses following the course of Isoniazid were resistant to this drug. Among 17 relapses in the control group, none were resistant(69). Thirdly, there is a definite need for close supervision with a consequent strain on health services. This supervision is necessary not only because of the slight danger of toxicity, but above all in order to ensure compliance. The disadvantage of placing too great a strain on health services by chemoprophylaxis program was well illustrated in the Canadian North where large number of native people were placed on a chemoprophylactic regimen. In consequence, in some areas the same degree of effort was placed on keeping individuals on prophylaxis as was placed on keeping active cases on treatment. The health personnel in some areas did not realize that treatment is much more important than prophylaxis; consequently the effort spent on supervision of treatment suffered. Finally, we have come to the somewhat ridiculous situation in which the duration of chemotherapy for active, even advanced, tuberculosis is shorter than the duration of the course of chemoprophylaxis. INH-chemoprophylaxis to be adequate is usually given for one year whereas treatment of even the advanced cases is being reduced to nine months. Reduction of chemoprophylaxis to say six months would give us diminished effectiveness, shown at least in the trial on fibrotic lesions in Eastern Europe but it may be wise to settle for shorter duration even if slightly less effective.

The discussion above related to giving INH prophylaxis to subjects already infected with tubercle bacilli; this is sometimes called secondary chemoprophylaxis. What about giving Isoniazid to the uninfected tuberculin negative individuals—so-called primary chemoprophylaxis? With very rare exceptions, primary chemoprophylaxis in the author's judgement should not be used. Some authorities recommend giving Isoniazid to all children, contacts of active cases, irrespective of the result of tuberculin reaction. As has already been discussed, tuberculosis is not a very infectious disease and even the smear positive cases only manage to infect about one third of the children contacts. The time when these become infected is unknown but they have probably been infected during a period of at least a few months in an average tuberculous household. When one sees a tuberculin negative child at the first contact examination, there is of course the possibility that this child had been infected, but is being examined during the incubation period, before tuberculin conversion. If that is the case, then we will know soon enough, as on retesting in six weeks' time his reaction will become positive. Although there is no real hard data on this point, in the author's experience the number of such children who become positive on second test is small. It is of course also possible for a child to be infected after the source was diagnosed and placed on chemotherapy, but this is unlikely as infectivity diminishes rapidly, and the patient knowing that he or she has tuberculosis takes appropriate precautions against infecting his children. The author used primary chemoprophylaxis on only one occasion in the case of two tuberculin negative infants, whose mother had extensive tuberculosis but refused admission to hospital and was thought likely to be noncompliant with treatment.

The mechanism of action of chemoprophylaxis is probably the same as it is of chemotherapy—namely the diminution of the bacterial population in the body.

What then are the indications for chemoprophylaxis? They are obviously situations with high-risk of development of tuberculous disease. Chemoprophylaxis should be given to:

1) Tuberculin positive contacts of cases of active tuberculosis particularly children and young adults up to the age of 35. Occasionally, the author does not recommend chemoprophylaxis in young adults, if they come from an area in which tuberculous infection is still very

common and positive reaction is likely to have been acquired in childhood. (e.g., immigrants from high-prevalence countries). In contacts, the "positive" reaction should include any reaction over 5 mm to 5 T.U.'s of PPD.

2) Inactive cases of tuberculosis under the age of 45 who did not receive adequate chemotherapy in the past. With the passage of time the number of such cases becomes progressively smaller. Individuals with fibrotic lesions (radiological shadow suggestive of healed post-primary pulmonary tuberculosis with positive tuberculin reaction) should also be treated.

3) Special indication: these are individuals with positive tuberculin reactions and radiological abnormalities subjected to special risk factors, particularly those placed on prolonged corticosteroid therapy. Younger silicotics, infected individuals undergoing gastrectomy and infected juvenile diabetics form other groups justifying chemoprophylaxis.

When chemoprophylaxis is limited to these indications, the number of individuals placed on preventive treatment in a given area will be roughly equal or only slightly greater than the number of those treated for active tuberculosis. This one-to-one ratio between chemoprophylaxis and treatment is probably optimal, and at least in Canada the areas which grossly exceed this ratio probably overuse, and those in which this ratio is less than 1 to 1 probably underutilize, this valuable program.

Isoniazid alone given for a period of 6–12 months should constitute the standard course of chemoprophylaxis although occasionally in selected cases with quite extensive radiological shadows, the author uses a two drug regimen. It must be emphasized that active tuberculosis must always be excluded by appropriate investigations, particularly by bacteriological studies before INH alone is given. As the results of cultures take several weeks to come back, the author often starts chemoprophylaxis with two drugs and then when cultures are reported to be negative switches to Isoniazid alone.

A chemoprophylactic program is not of sufficiently high priority to be adopted in developing countries, until the treatment program is running very satisfactorily. This is not to say that chemoprophylaxis may not be practised in clinical medicine in those countries when indication exists, it would be a mistake however to make it a part of the national program and thus dilute the effort directed toward treatment.

Should drugs other than INH be utilized in chemoprophylaxis when the source case harbours INH-resistant bacilli? The answer to this fortunately uncommon problem is difficult, but should probably, in the present stage of our knowledge, be negative. Contacts infected by INH-resistant cases should, however, be carefully watched for years.

CONCLUSIONS

Tuberculosis in most countries of the world is in the state of steady but slow decline. The rate of this decline can be accelerated by well conceived tuberculosis programs. Unfortunately it can also be retarded by a poor program for instance when poor treatment results in large number of "program produced chronics."

In many developed countries, tuberculosis rates are already so low that special tuberculosis services, which have done so much for tuberculosis in the past are being gradually phased out. Tuberculosis is, therefore, returning into the mainstream of medicine with respirologists, infectious disease specialists, internists, general physicians, etc., increasingly looking after rising proportion of tuberculous patients. Yet, the general level of professional education and of awareness of tuberculosis is unfortunately rather low in North America and various health professionals are not yet quite ready to assume effective responsibility for tuberculosis. While the disease is relatively uncommon today, it is much more frequent than most health professionals appear to assume. A major educational effort is therefore needed.

In many developing countries, rates of tuberculosis are still very high, and the size of the problem is so large, that general public health approaches are essential. They include diagnosis by sputum microscopy and standardized chemotherapy delivered by peripheral health personnel. It is in the area of treatment that greater emphasis should be placed as the results are poor.

Case finding and treatment programs remain the backbone of prevention of tuberculosis. Two specific preventive programs, BCG vaccination and chemoprophylaxis are capable of making a more modest but nevertheless substantial contribution. Curiously, it is infrequent for any single country to use both programs simultaneously in an efficient way. There is no real rivalry between BCG vaccination and chemoprophylaxis, the first being used among tuberculin negative uninfected individuals, whereas the second is used almost entirely in those already infected. The best results from the preventive programs will be achieved by their concurrent but circumscribed use.

REFERENCES

1. Grzybowski S., Barnett G.D., Styblo K. (1975) Contacts of cases of active pulmonary tuberculosis. Selected Papers *16:* 90 Royal Netherlands Tuberculosis Association
2. Riley R.L. (1967) The hazard is relative. Amer Rev Res Dis *96:* 623
3. Chan-Yeung M., Galbraith J.D., Schulson N., Brown A., Grzybowski S. (1971) Reactivation of inactive tuberculosis in northern Canada. Amer Rev Res Dis *104:*861
4. Nakielna E.M., Cragg R., Grzybowski S. (1975) Life long follow-up of inactive tuberculosis: its value and limitation. Amer Rev Res Dis *112:*765
5. NissenMeyer S. (1949) *Statistical Investigations of the Relationship of Tuberculosis Morbidity and Mortality to Infection.* E. Munksgaard, Copenhagen
6. Stead W.W. (1952) Personal Communication
7. Grzybowski S., Allen E.A. (1964) The challenge of tuberculosis in decline. Amer Rev Res Dis *90:*51
8. Bentley F.J., Grzybowski S., Benjamin B. (1954) *Tuberculosis in Childhood and Adolescence.* National Association for the Prevention of Tuberculosis, London
9. Wallgren A. (1948) The time table of tuberculosis. Tubercle *29:*245
10. Galbraith J.D., Grzybowski S., Law C.L., Rowe J.F. (1969) Tuberculosis in Indian children: primary pulmonary tuberculosis. Can Med Assoc J *11:*497
11. Daniels M., Ridehalgh F., Springett V.H., Hall I.M. (1948) *Tuberculosis in Young Adults. Report on the Prophit Tuberculosis Survey 1935: 1944.* H.K. Lewis, London
12. Ustvedt H.J. (1947) Further investigations concerning relation between erythema nodosum and tuberculosis. Tubercle *28:*247

13. Eliasberg H., Neuland W. (1921) Die epituberkulose Infiltration der Lunge bei tuberkulosen Sauglingen und Kindern. Jahrb. f. Kinderheilk *94:*102
14. Brock R.C. (1950) Post-tuberculous bronchostenosis and bronchiectasis in the middle lobe. Thorax *5:*5
15. Nathhorst H. (1948) The prognosis of exudative pleurisy in children. Acta tuberc Scand suppl 17
16. Enarson D.A., Ashley M.J., Grzybowski S. (1979) Tuberculosis in immigrants to Canada. Amer Rev Res Dis *119:*11
17. Schvira V. (1959) Experience with pericarditis at H. Grote-Schuur Hospital, Capetown. S A Med Journal *33:*810
18. Marfan A. (1886) De l'immunite conferee par la guerison d'une tuberculose locale pour la phthisie pulmonaire. Arch. gen. de Med. *57:*575
19. Enarson D.A., Fujii M., Nakielna E.M., Grzybowski S. (1979) Bone and joint tuberculosis: a continuing problem. Can Med Assoc J *120:*139
20. Medical Research Council Working Party on Tuberculosis of the Spine, Seventh Report (1978). Tubercle *59:*79
21. Simon G. (1930) Sekundāre Streuherde der Lunge, insbesondere der frühen Spitzenherde. *Engel-Pirquet Hdbch. d. Kindertuberk,* Leipzig
22. Grzybowski S., Dorken E., Bates C. (1969) Disparities of tuberculin. Amer Rev Res Dis *100:*86
23. Hamman L., Wilman S. (1912) *Tuberculin in Diagnosis and Treatment.* D Appleton and Co., New York
24. Styblo K. (1970) Transmission of tuberculous infection; other results of the work of the Tuberculosis Surveillance Research Unit (TSRU). Bull Int Un. Tuberc *43:*95
25. Meijer J. (1970) Possible consequences of TSRU's findings on antituberculosis programmes in low prevalence countries. Bull Int Un. Tuberc *43:*106
26. Brink G.C., Grzybowski S., Lane G.B. (1960) Silicotuberculosis. Can Med Assoc J *82:*959
27. Olin J.S., Grzybowski S. (1966) Tuberculosis and Alcoholism. Can Med Assoc J *94:*999
28. Crofton J., Douglas A. (1975) *Respiratory Diseases 2nd Ed.* Blackwell Scientific Publications, Oxford, p 200
29. Grzybowski S., McKinnon N.E., Tuters L., Pinkus G., Philipps R. (1966) Reactivations in inactive pulmonary tuberculosis. Amer Rev Res Dis *93:*352
30. National Tuberculosis Institute, Bangalore (1974) Tuberculosis in a rural population of South India: a five year epidemiological study. Bull Wld Hlth Org *51:*473.

supervised twice-weekly regimen of chemotherapy in a routine out-patient treatment programme. Ind J Tuberc *21:*152
31. Springett V.H. (1971) Ten year results during the introduction of chemotherapy for tuberculosis. Tubercle *52:*73
32. Rutledge C.J.A., Cronch J.B. (1919) The ultimate results in 1,694 cases of tuberculosis treated at the Modern Woodmen of America Sanatorium. Amer Rev Tuberc *2:*755–763
33. Jang K. (1979) A comparative evaluation of hospital versus clinic education of tuberculosis patients in Vancouver. MSc Thesis. University of British Columbia
34. Dutt A.K., Stead W.W. (1981) Chemotherapy of tuberculosis for the 1980's. Clinics in Chest Medicine Vol 243
35. Kopanoff D.E., Snider D.E. Jr., Caras G.J. (1978) Isoniazid related hepatitis. Amer Rev Res Dis *117:*991
36. Edwards L.B., Palmer C.E. (1958) Epidemiologic studies of tuberculin sensitivity: I Preliminary results with purified protein derivatives prepared from atypical acid-fast organisms. Amer J Hyg *68:*213
37. U.S. Public Health Service: *A Child Centered Program to Prevent Tuberculosis.* Publication No 1280, Washington
38. Grzybowski S., Brown M., Stothard D. (1969) Infections with atypical mycobacteria in British Columbia. Can Med Assoc J *100:*869
39. Narain R., Anantharaman D.S., Diwakara A.M. (1974) Prevalence of non-specific tuberculin sensitivity in certain parts of India. Bull Wld Hlth Org *51:*273
40. Edwards L.B., Palmer C.E., Comstock G.W. (1968) Contributions of northern populations to the understanding of tuberculin sensitivity. Arch Environ Hlth *17:*507
41. Edwards L.B., Hopwood L., Palmer C.E. (1965) Identification of mycobacterial infections. Bull Wld Hlth Org *33:*405
42. Grzybowski S. (1963) Testing the tuberculin test. Canada's Health and Welfare *18:*(5) 4
43. Grzybowski S. (1951) Tuberculin sensitivity in children suffering from pulmonary tuberculosis. Tubercle *32:*145
44. Comstock G.W., Edwards L.B., Philip R.N., Winn W.A. (1964) A comparison in the United States of America of two tuberculins PPD-S and RT_{23}. Bull Wld Hlth Org *31:*161
45. American Thoracic Society Committee on Diagnostic Skin Testing (1971). Amer Rev Res Dis *104:*769
46. Grzybowski S., Kincade G., McLean C.C., Rowe J.F. (1968) Size of tuberculin reactions in various age groups. Amer Rev Res Dis *98:*303

47. Complementary document (1965) "Results of the multiple radiophotography reading trial performed in 1963." Bull Int Un Tuberc *36:*61
48. Cruickshank D.B. (1952) *Bacteriology of Tuberculosis in Modern Practise of Tuberculosis.* Sellars T.H. and Livingstone J.L. eds, Butterworth, London
49. Chandrasekhar P., Nair S.S., Ras P.K., Rao G.R., Pyarelal (1970) Examination of multiple sputum specimens in a tuberculosis survey. Tuberc *51:*255
50. Devadatta A., Radhakrishna S., Fox W., Mitchison D.A., Rajogopalan S. Sivasubranamian, Stott H. (1966) Comparative value of sputum smear examination and culture examination in assessing the progress of tuberculous patients receiving chemotherapy. Bull Wld Hltc Org *34:*573
51. Phillips P.A., Pinkus G. (1976) Sputum conversion in Eskimos. Tubercle *57* (4) Supplement 51
52. Fox W., Mitchison D.A. (1975) Short course chemotherapy for pulmonary tuberculosis. Amer Rev Res Dis *111:*325
53. Grzybowski S., Marr W.B. (1963) The unchanging pattern of pulmonary tuberculosis. Can Med Assoc J *89:*741
54. Enarson D.A., Sjögren I., Grzybowski S. (1980) Incidence of tuberculosis among Scandinavian immigrants in Canada. Scand J Res Dis *61:*139–142
55. Grzybowski S. (1965) Ontario studies on tuberculin sensitivity. Can J Pub Hlth *56:*181
56. Grzybowski S., Brown M.T., Rowe J.F. (1969) Significance of the tuberculin reaction. Can Med Assoc J *100:*984
57. Palmer C.E., Long M.W. (1966) Effects of infection with atypical mycobacteria on BCG vaccination and tuberculosis. Amer Rev Res Dis *94:*553
58. Robakiewicz M., Grzybowski S. (1974) Epidemiologic aspects of nontuberculous mycobacterial disease and of tuberculosis in British Columbia. Amer Rev Res Dis *109:*613
59. Chai H Ahn., Hurst George A. (1981) The Treatment of Mycobacterium Avium-Intracellulare Complex Disease. Seminars in Respiratory Medicine Vol 2 233
60. Dutt A.K., Stead W.W. (1979) Long term results of medical treatment in mycobacterium intracellulare infections. Amer J of Med *67:*449
61. Myers J.A. (1957) A summary of the views opposing BCG. Adv Tuberc Res *8:*272

62. Sutherland I. (1972) State of the art in immunoprophylaxis in tuberculosis *in Immunization in Tuberculosis,* E.C. Chamberlayne ed. Forgarty International Center Proceedings No 14, Washington 113
63. Tuberculosis Prevention Trial, Madras. (1980) Trial of BCG vaccines in south India for tuberculosis prevention. Indian J Med Res *72* (Suppl) p. 1–74
64. Grzybowski S. (1972) BCG in developing versus developed countries *in Immunization in Tuberculosis* E.C. Chanberlayne ed. Fogarty International Centre Proceedings No 14, Washington 127
65. Ferebee S.H. (1970) Controlled chemoprophylaxis trials in tuberculosis—a general review. Adv. Tuberc Res *17:*28
66. Krebs A. (1976) The IUAT trial on isoniazid preventive treatment in persons with fibrotic lung lesions. Bull Int Un Tuberc *51:*193
67. Grzybowski S., Ashley M.J., McKinnon N.E., Pinkus G., Philipps R., Brown A. (1969) In Canada: a trial of chemoprophylaxis in inactive tuberculosis. Can Med Assoc J. *101:*555
68. Grzybowski S., Styblo K., Dorken E. (1976) Tuberculosis in Eskimos. Tubercle *57:*(4) Supplement
69. Grzybowski S., Ashley M.J., Pinkus G. (1976) Chemoprophylaxis in inactive tuberculosis: long term evaluation of a Canadian trial. Can Med Assoc J *114:*607
70. Levin M.L., Moodie A.S. (1976) Isoniazid prophylaxis and deaths in Baltimore, Maryland 1972. Bull Int Un Tuberc *51:*213
71. Grzybowski S., Enarson D.A. (1978) The Fate of Cases of Pulmonary Tuberculosis under various treatment programmes. Bull Int Un Tuberc *53:*70
72. Ferguson R.G. (1955) *Studies in Tuberculosis,* Toronto. Univ of Toronto Press 97
73. Fox W. (1981) Whither short-course chemotherapy? Br J Dis Chest *75:*331.
74. Edwards L.B., Acquaviva F.A., Livesay V.T. (1973) Identification of tuberculous infected: dual tests of density and reaction. Amer Rev Res Dis *18:*1334.
75. Grzybowski S., Galbraith J.D., Dorken E. (1976) Chemoprophylaxis trial in Canadian Eskimos. Tubercle *57:*263.

INDEX